probiotics
for Crohn's & Colitis

by

PETER CARTWRIGHT

To my wife, Yvonne,
without whose prayers and support
this book would not have been possible.

D0227362

Published by
Prentice Publishing
PO Box 1704
Ilford IG5 0WN
United Kingdom
Tel/fax: +44 (0)20 8551 6192
mail@prentice-publishing.co.uk
www.prentice-publishing.co.uk

Printed and bound in Great Britain by
Antony Rowe Ltd., Chippenham, Wiltshire

A CIP record for this publication
is available from the British Library

ISBN 0-9544438-0-2

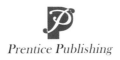

Prentice Publishing

Contents

Foreword 5

Testimonials 7

1. Introduction 9

2. The History of Probiotics 17

3. IBD, Bacteria & Inflammation 33

4. Probiotics for IBD: Evidence for benefits 46

5. Specific Species & Strains 54

6. Prebiotics –What Are They? 69

7. Specific Prebiotics 77

8. Other Benefits of Probiotics 87

9. Questions & Answers on Probiotics 96

Appendix 1: The Body's Defence Systems 103

Appendix 2: Safety of Probiotics 108

References 118

Index 127

Acknowledgements

A lot of people have helped me with this book. Of particular note is medical journalist Sara M. Bernstein, formerly of the Crohn's and Colitis Foundation of America. In skilfully editing this book she made crucial suggestions on restructuring which improved the text very substantially.

If Sara was my scientific editor, Loulou Brown was my literary editor. Her recommendations cut out most of the waffle, made the messages far clearer, and avoided excessive jargon.

Among my colleagues and friends at the National Association for Colitis and Crohn's Disease (NACC), Christine Bertoloni, Deirdre Choo, Sarah Masters and Stephanie Sadler were all most encouraging, and provided knowledgeable commentary on likely readership response.

Substantial guidance has been given to me by a number of gastroenterologists and scientists. In addition to those who provided quoted testimonials, supportive comments were received from Professors Derek Jewell, John Hunter and Jonathan Rhodes, and from Drs Roy Fuller and Stephen Grainger.

Staff from several probiotic companies have also been very helpful in clarifying details about their own products and related matters.

The following NACC members gave me information about their experiences with probiotics: Aileen Aldred, Mr and Mrs K. Banks, Mrs Diana Bartlett, Alison Brooks, David Clarke, Sue Clements, Arash Dabestani, Bob Davies, Harry Edwards, Jill Eldridge, Karen Erlebach, Kathleen Harper, Mary Hender, Michelle Hendry, Ann Holmes, Sheila King, Anthea Mander Lahr, Russell Marsh, Ian Matheson, Stuart McLean, Adrian Miller, Bill Murray, Miss Gillian Packington, Sue Perrin, Chris Polhill, Harriet Powell, Mr Norman Seal, David Sharman, Miss Gina Sparks, Mrs Clara Steels, David Taggart, Ann Thorne, Mr Michael Truscott and Mr Gerald Woods.

The convivial and knowledgeable Havering Writers' Circle gave me the opportunity to read sections of the text before an audience. This was an excellent way of testing whether my writing was fluent and understandable.

Gillian Oliver (illustrator), Paul Jones (cover design) and George Mann (layout and production) all used their talents to the substantial benefit of this book.

Thank you to everyone listed above, and my apologies to anyone I have accidentally omitted.

Foreword

The contents of the human gut represent an enormously complex ecosystem comprising huge numbers and highly varied populations of bacteria. This living mass of bacteria is tantamount to a virtual, hidden organ within each of us. Generally, the intestinal bacteria are an asset to health maintenance, but occasionally, in susceptible individuals, some of the bacteria may become a potential liability. Scientists are now beginning to study how to promote these bacterial assets and how to offset potential liabilities.

The commonest demonstration of the role of intestinal bacteria in health maintenance is the development of abdominal symptoms (and sometimes serious disease) when intestinal bacteria are disturbed by consumption of broad-spectrum antibiotics. On the other hand, perhaps the best example of bacterial involvement in causing intestinal disease has been the discovery that bacteria within the stomach of some individuals (*Helicobacter pylori*) can cause ulcers. This served a sobering lesson for scientists and allayed much of the scepticism relating to the participation of resident intestinal bacteria in chronic disease. More recently, attention has been directed at the potential role of bacteria in diseases such as Crohn's, colitis and colorectal cancer. Fortunately, one can fight fire with fire, and some of the intestinal bacteria can be used as preventive or treatment strategies. For example, several types of bacteria within the human gut can compete against harmful or pathogenic bacteria and can have anti-inflammatory effects. This means they can be used as probiotics. The definition of probiotics is undergoing continual refinement but they can be operationally described as gut bacteria, which have beneficial properties that can be exploited for health promotion or disease treatment.

Although the causes of Crohn's and colitis are not known, these diseases appear to involve an interplay amongst three contributory elements: genes, immunity and bacteria. We can do nothing about our genetic constitution, and treatments for inflammatory bowel disease have generally fallen into the category of suppressors or modifiers of the immune and inflammatory responses. However, the contribution of intestinal bacteria has, until recently, received little attention as a therapeutic opportunity. Because of the side effects and toxicity of many of the anti-inflammatory and immunosuppressant drugs, there is a need to exploit safer strategies geared toward manipulation of the gut flora. This, in essence, is the principle behind the use of probiotics in Crohn's and colitis.

Can we make sense of the deluge of scientific data on gut bacteria and probiotics? We must be wary of enthusiasts and faddists and distinguish fact from fiction. What is the quality of the evidence for probiotics in inflammatory bowel disease? The patient as a consumer needs a sound and simple explanation of the area. I am delighted to be able to state that Peter Cartwright has succeeded in providing a balanced perspective on the field with a crisp, lucid and readable account that is both concise and sufficiently comprehensive.

Probiotics may emerge either as functional food ingredients or as pharmabiotic drugs. Whatever their regulatory designation, their potential has yet to be realised and requires continuing scientific scrutiny. Peter Cartwright's account will be a useful primer to provide background perspective and enable patients and other consumers to judge the strength and relevance of the evidence as it unfolds over the next decade.

Fergus Shanahan, M.D.,

Department of Medicine,
University College Cork,
National University of Ireland,
Cork.

Testimonials

Peter Cartwright has written a clear and authoritative explanation, which will help many patients to understand this new approach to the treatment of IBD ~ **Richard Driscoll, Director, National Association for Colitis and Crohn's Disease, U.K.**

This is a readily comprehensible book and a welcome addition to the literature – a 'must read' for colitis patients and their families ~ **G.T. Macfarlane, Professor of Bacteriology, University of Dundee, Scotland.**

An ideal book on medical information is one that can be enjoyed both by patients and medical practitioners. This book on probiotics for Crohn's and colitis is full of accurate information both for patients and doctors and covers a most exciting area of rapid medical advance. It captures very well the promises and uncertainties ~ **Professor Subrata Ghosh, Imperial College London, Hammersmith Hospital.**

This book is an important document and meets a great need. I hope that it will popularize the use of natural biological treatments and help numerous patients suffering from IBD to control their disease ~ **Stig Bengmark M.D., Honorary Visiting Professor, Departments of Hepatology and Surgery, University College, London.**

IBD is a major cause of medical suffering and patients should be supported as much as possible. New findings in the area of probiotics and prebiotics offer much hope and opportunity in alleviating symptoms, however the research is disparate. Here, Peter Cartwright has done a first class job of pulling together all the relevant information into one volume. There are valuable insights into the products that offer the best chances of success and mechanisms of effect are explained in a clear and thoughtful manner. It is hoped that new inroads into IBD treatment and prevention may result from probiotic and prebiotic use. Thus, the book will be extremely useful for sufferers as well as their care staff. It will also greatly interest those who are generally interested in the use of dietary intervention and gastrointestinal disorder ~ **Professor G. R. Gibson, Food Microbial Sciences Unit, School of Biosciences, University of Reading, England.**

The use of bacteria to help alleviate inflammatory bowel disease may seem a bizarre concept, both to laymen and many medical practitioners. However, as explained clearly and concisely by Peter Cartwright, the scientific principles and practical results fully justify the growing optimism for this novel method of management. I am happy to recommend this book not only to sufferers from inflammatory bowel disease but also to a wider audience, including dieticians, general practitioners and gastroenterologists ~ **Jeremy Hamilton-Miller, Professor of Medical Microbiology, Royal Free and University College Medical School, London.**

Nothing is more appealing to patients than the idea of being treated with safe and effective 'natural products'. While this remains a dream for most serious illnesses, emerging evidence suggests that some forms of chronic gut inflammation, like Crohn's disease, ulcerative colitis and pouchitis, may be amenable to therapy based on 'friendly bacteria' (probiotics) or foodstuff (prebiotics) that fosters their growth. This book provides comprehensive, evidence-based information that probiotics and prebiotics may become part of the therapeutic armamentarium for inflammatory bowel diseases in the near future ~ **Claudio Fiocchi, Professor of Medicine, Case Western Reserve University, Cleveland, U.S.A.**

'Probiotics for Crohn's and Colitis' forms an important new guidebook for people suffering from these disorders. Probiotics have a long history of use, but the science behind them has been mostly accumulated during the last decade. Old beliefs in the use of lactic acid bacteria and bifidobacteria have finally been proved right. The specific strains, usually isolated from the healthy infant or adult intestinal microbiota, form the new generation of well-defined and documented probiotic bacteria.

I feel strongly that the time has come to apply the knowledge on probiotics to clinical practice. Mr Cartwright has done an excellent job in exploring and summarizing the evidence. This will provide practical science-based guidance for the use of probiotics in dietary management of IBD. Coupled with medical information and practice this book is an excellent source of information to assist in selecting the individual probiotics for specific symptoms ~ **Professor Seppo Salminen, Program on Health Bioscience, University of Turku, Finland.**

1. Introduction

"I have had UC for 26 years and used to feel permanently bloated, had awful wind and a very 'gurgling' stomach. About every two weeks, I used to get bad stomach ache and the runs. I started taking a probiotic milk drink, and felt the benefits after 3 days. Now I feel more or less normal. While on holiday and unable to obtain the probiotic drink, the above problems recur – fortunately vanishing within a few days of starting to take it again."

The purpose of this book is to explain how some bacteria, taken in food or as supplements, can probably help reduce the severity of Crohn's Disease or Ulcerative Colitis (UC). The products that contain these beneficial bacteria are called **probiotics**, and the bacteria that have health-improving effects are called probiotic bacteria.

The probiotic bacteria have an effect upon the microflora (the billions of bacteria that live in the intestines of every human being, also known as gut bacteria). The microflora, through their normal living processes, have a range of effects on the health of their host. These effects may be negative or positive depending on a range of factors, including the type and numbers of bacteria that constitute the microflora at a particular time.

The value of probiotics is that, by being consumed as food or as supplements, they can alter the microflora and increase the likelihood that the overall effect of the gut bacterial processes is health improvement rather than health deterioration.

The health improvements that arise from taking probiotics affect those diseases influenced by the microflora, and prominent among those diseases are Crohn's and UC.

The effect of probiotics on Crohn's and UC

Much is still unknown about the bacteria in the human gut, and the exact causes of Crohn's and UC are not yet known. Despite this incomplete picture, however, there is growing scientific evidence that probiotic bacteria may constitute a significant breakthrough in the treatment of Inflammatory Bowel Disease (IBD), which is the collective name used for UC and Crohn's.

Scientific evidence suggests that by increasing the numbers of these beneficial bacteria in your small intestine and colon you may be able to:

- reduce the severity of a flare-up,
- lengthen the time that the disease stays in remission, and
- strengthen your immune system.

Probiotics may enable people with IBD to reduce prescribed drugs and, as a consequence, the side effects caused by these drugs. Furthermore, by reducing the severity of the disease, it may be possible to postpone surgery or even avoid it altogether.

Perhaps this sounds too good to be true; that here is yet another writer making extravagant claims and exploiting people's anxieties about a very unpleasant long-term condition. Nevertheless, this book is based on scientific evidence, written in ordinary English, and it should enable you to judge for yourself the evidence in favour of probiotics.

This book also explains the scientific theories of how probiotic bacteria appear to work, and provides general guidance on probiotic products.

There is also information about **prebiotics,** which are types of soluble carbohydrate that encourage the growth of beneficial bacteria. This word will be written as '*pre*biotics' in this book, with an italicised prefix, to make it easier to distinguish from 'probiotics'.

Reasons for reading this book

If you have IBD, you may not want to spend time reading a book about probiotics; instead you may wish to start taking probiotics and see whether they have any positive effects. You may even have tried probiotics already.

I would strongly recommend reading this book for three reasons:

- IBD can be a serious condition and it is important to work with your doctor on this, if at all possible. The more knowledge you have about probiotics, the more confident you will be in speaking with your doctor and other members of the healthcare team;

- Not all probiotic bacteria will be effective with UC and Crohn's and it will be helpful to know what evidence there is about specific species and strains;

- Probiotic products vary considerably in their form and content, particularly in the numbers of live bacteria contained. This book gives information on the main factors you should be looking for in a suitable product.

How reliable is the information?

The information on probiotics contained in this book is based on reliable research as recorded in scientific journals and specialist texts. Sources of this information are given in a list of references towards the end of the book. If you or your doctor wish to investigate a particular aspect in greater detail, there are some leads to follow.

In reporting on research into probiotics, I have concentrated on major research journals, mainly in the fields of gastroenterology, microbiology and nutrition. Also, in clinical trials I distinguish between small studies and randomised controlled trials (RCTs).

RCTs involve large numbers of participants and more statistical techniques to help ensure that the results are a true record of cause and effect. Also, these studies involve control groups; one group of participants receives the treatment and a similar 'control' group remains untreated, enabling the results to be more accurately assessed for bias.

If a reported study has a low number of participants or lacks a control group, I try to point this out. This is so that you are in a better position to judge the strength of the evidence.

Where do bacteria fit into the picture of IBD?

The continuing or recurrent inflammation of the intestines of people with UC and Crohn's is believed to involve several factors. Among these are genes, the malfunctioning of the immune system and the microflora. It is not known, however, exactly how these elements interact to cause IBD.

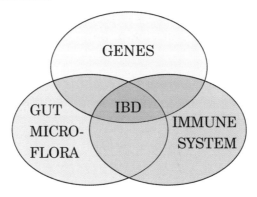

Fig 1 – Three main factors involved in IBD

In the treatment of IBD, prescribed drugs have helped significantly to bring the disease under control. In particular, drugs have reduced the risk of death to a very low level – something that used to be a real threat in severe cases. But these drugs have their limitations (they do not work on everyone with IBD; they may have side effects), and so the search for improved treatments continues.

Diet is increasingly considered an integral part of IBD care. For example, liquid elemental drinks are given to teenagers to improve their weight and possibly reduce the need for strong drugs; and some adults may have reduced symptoms by removing certain foods from their diet if they are intolerant to them.

Until relatively recently, the microflora were thought to be of little importance in the cause of IBD, and, therefore, alteration of the types of bacteria that make up the microflora had not been considered seriously as a treatment. Over the last twenty years, however, enough evidence has been obtained to suggest that not only are microflora important for the continuation of the disease, but also that certain types of beneficial bacteria may be used in treatment.

In summary, while much remains unknown about IBD, it is increasingly clear that gut bacteria are a factor in the disease and that probiotic bacteria may be able to play a role in breaking the cycle of IBD inflammation. The role of these probiotic bacteria will be explained in this book.

Aren't all bacteria harmful?

The popular image of bacteria is as a disease-causing enemy that should be killed at every opportunity. Each home contains anti-bacterial products to keep disease at bay.

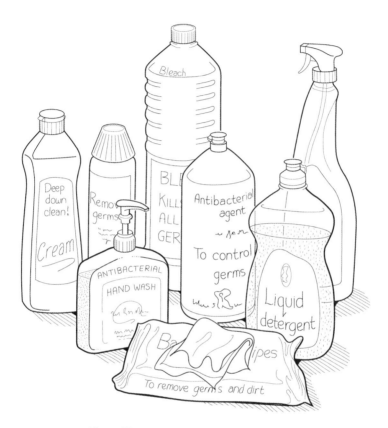

Fig 2. Household anti-bacterial products

Probiotic products contain millions, even billions, of bacteria, so it is not unreasonable to question whether probiotics are safe.

There are bacteria that are responsible for many severe infectious diseases such as tuberculosis, diphtheria, cholera, typhoid, tetanus and leprosy. But there are many different types of bacteria; some are harmful to humans, and some are helpful. Most are neutral, but may be harmful depending on particular circumstances.

The bacteria used in probiotics, mostly those that produce lactic acid, are very safe but no bacterium is completely safe. There is always the possibility, no matter how slight, that any bacteria will behave in an unexpected and harmful manner. However, probiotic bacteria very rarely cause harm, and it is virtually unknown for harm to come from probiotic products.

The subject of safety is covered more fully in chapter 5, as well as in Appendix 2.

Structure of the book

The structure of this book has been planned to help people with Crohn's or UC, together with their spouses, partners, close relatives or friends, to understand the option of probiotics (and *pre*biotics).

Each chapter is introduced by a quote from a person with IBD who takes probiotics regularly. The intention is to share personal experiences and show that there are people with IBD who appear to benefit from probiotics. The quotes were drawn from replies to a notice in the newsletter of the National Association for Colitis and Crohn's Disease requesting experiences with probiotics, 'good, bad, or indifferent'. Of the 33 replies, two people doubted they had had any benefit and another stopped taking a probiotic milk drink after she developed an allergic reaction (blotchy red skin and severe itching). All the rest were very positive about the probiotics they use. One should not assume, however, that all products that describe themselves as probiotic will necessarily benefit a person with IBD.

Chapter **2** looks at the history of probiotics. It shows that:

- foods produced with the use of bacteria have been consumed safely for thousands of years;
- scientific support for the idea of consuming beneficial bacteria (in the form of fermented milks) to improve health is about a hundred years old;
- fermented milks lost their popularity following criticism of unsubstantiated claims; and
- the idea of probiotics, the modern term for beneficial bacterial products, became very popular over the last decade of the twentieth century.

It is to be hoped that Chapter **2** will provide some reassurance that probiotics are not merely a passing fad and that they have historical substance.

Chapter **3** describes how IBD is believed to develop, including the role of bacteria and the importance of the immune system. This should make it clear why finding a cure has proved so elusive, and how bacteria might play a very important role. This chapter also refers to an Appendix 1, which explains the body's defence systems more fully.

Chapter **4** looks in some detail at the evidence for the use of probiotics in IBD. The method used is to draw upon eight 'research reviews' by leading experts, and report on the key studies.

Chapter **5** looks at specific probiotic bacteria (and yeasts) and assesses, with each type, what evidence there is for any beneficial effect. If you are considering the ingredients of a probiotic product, the information provided in this chapter will enable you to check whether any reliable scientific evidence backs up the listed bacteria.

The following two chapters, **6** and **7**, look at *pre*biotics. These are non-digestible food ingredients that provide nutrients for beneficial bacteria. When *pre*biotics are consumed, the desirable bacteria that are already present in the intestines tend to grow in numbers, at the expense of harmful bacteria. The *pre*biotic approach to manipulating the microflora is therefore different from the probiotic approach (working on existing gut bacteria, rather than adding new ones). Probiotic products can also contain *pre*biotics, to help the probiotic bacteria to grow within the human intestine.

Chapter **8** describes how probiotics and prebiotics may help other intestinal conditions, which may also affect people with IBD.

The final chapter, **9**, contains questions and answers, which reinforce the main points of the book and discusses practical matters. Information is also provided about possible future developments.

At the end of each chapter there is a summary of the main points, to help the reader absorb and retain the information provided.

Further information, and a list of IBD Associations in different countries, can be found on the publisher's web site (www.prentice-publishing.co.uk).

Chapter summary

- Probiotics, containing beneficial bacteria, can probably help reduce the severity of Crohn's and UC.

- The information in this book will help you to discuss probiotics with your doctor, learn about different species and strains of probiotic bacteria, and know what to look for when selecting a probiotic product.

- The book is based on scientific evidence, and is written in straightforward English for the general reader.

- Along with genes and the immune system, the microflora (gut bacteria) are involved in IBD inflammation. Probiotics aim to alter the microflora so that the inflammation is reduced, and periods of remission extended.

- *Pre*biotics alter the microflora by providing 'food' that is favoured by beneficial bacteria that are already living in the gut.

- Unlike many other types of bacteria, probiotic bacteria (mostly lactic acid producers) are very safe.

- The list of chapters is best read in numerical order; however, if you wish to read them out of order, it makes sense to read chapters 4 and 5 together, and 6 and 7 together.

2. The History of Probiotics

"Since taking a probiotic powder, containing a mixture of various lactobacilli and organically-grown plant materials, my life has been transformed. My Crohn's, which affects the terminal ileum and a small bit of the colon, has been in total remission for some 18 months. I no longer need to take steroids or mesalazine, and am in the process of slowly reducing azathioprine."

The probiotic concept of using bacteria to improve health is a hundred years old, and the use of fermented foods (which involve bacteria) has a much longer history.

The evidence of the benefits of probiotics for IBD is still growing, and we need to draw on the entire history of probiotics to help to understand their applicability to IBD and the possibility of their use as a treatment option.

Definition

The term 'probiotic' was first used in 1965,[1] but it was not until 1989 that there was a widely accepted definition: "A live microbial feed supplement which beneficially affects the host animal by improving its intestinal microbial balance".[2] The use of the word 'feed' shows that the early use of the term probiotics related to farmed animals.

Antibiotics are used to make farm animals healthier by killing harmful bacteria. If another way of making animals healthy is to feed them beneficial bacteria, the logical name for these had to be 'probiotics'.

Although the word probiotic was only coined a few decades ago, the use of bacteria for health purposes has a much longer history.

Fermented drinks and foods

Micro-organisms (also known as microbes) have been used in fermented food and drink for thousands of years and possibly before recorded time. Fermentation happens when bacteria break down plant and animal material, gaining energy and chemicals that enables them to grow and reproduce. Some plants can also ferment, such as yeast, which is a type of fungus. One of the products of yeast fermentation is alcohol. The process of fermentation has been known for centuries, even if the cause and the chemical reactions involved have not been understood until more recently.

Wine is the fermented juice of grapes. The fermentation occurs naturally when yeasts on the grape skin react with the juice when the skin breaks. Organised vine growing and wine production has taken place for more than 5,000 years, apparently starting in South-West Asia.[3]

The production of beer also involves a fermentation process and beer has been produced for at least 3,500 years, possibly originating in Mesopotamia (now Iran and Iraq).[4]

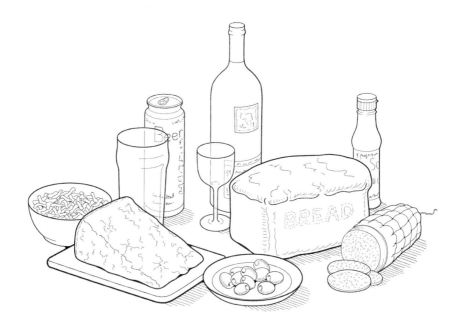

Fig 3. Fermented foods and drinks

2: The History of Probiotics

Various foods are made using fermentation. For instance, bread rises when the yeast ferments sugars in the dough and carbon dioxide is given off in tiny bubbles. Lactic acid bacteria are used to ferment sauerkraut (shredded cabbage), table olives, and European hard sausages (for example, salami) to preserve the food and improve the flavour. Soy sauce, from the Far East, is the product of fermented soya beans.

Many long-standing milk products involve fermentation. For example, there are 'soured milks' called *keffir* (Russia), *mazun* (Armenia), *gioddu* (Sardinia), *kumiss* (Asia), *leben* (Egypt), *dahi, lassi* (India) and yoghurt (the Balkans and Russia).

Traditional butter-making involved the cream being 'soured' before being churned. Cheese was originally developed by microbial fermentation in which the two parts of milk, the curd and the whey, were separated and the more solid curd (protein) formed the cheese. Adding other bacteria that form coloured veins develops flavours.

Humans have therefore used bacteria and yeasts for thousands of years to improve and preserve food. It is likely that these fermented foods first developed by accident, perhaps by Stone Age man burying food in the ground for safe keeping and finding that it was preserved as the result of natural fermentation.[5]

Bacteria first identified

The first person to see bacteria was a Dutch scientist, Antoni van Leeuwenhoek, in the seventeenth century. He reported to the Royal Society of London how, with the use of a primitive microscope, he had observed a wide range of 'animalcules' not normally visible to the human eye.[6]

But it was not until the middle of the nineteenth century that experimental methods and laboratory equipment improved sufficiently to enable a proper study of bacteria to take place.

During the latter half of the nineteenth century the French chemist Louis Pasteur showed that fermentation, as in wine production, was caused by micro-organisms. He also demonstrated that the decay of food into an inedible form was caused by micro-organisms and that the bad-smelling form of decay, putrefaction, was a type of fermentation.

Pasteur also developed the theory that microbes could cause disease. This was verified by various experiments conducted by other scientists in Europe.

Then, when the important French wine and vinegar industries were suffering from spoilage of their products, Pasteur solved the problem by developing a heat treatment. This process, later known as pasteurisation, killed off harmful bacteria, but did not spoil the product.

The colon: fermenting or putrefying?

At the turn of the twentieth century there was a debate in medicine about the significance of the huge numbers of bacteria in the human intestines, particularly the colon.

Was fermentation in the bowels good or bad? Were intestinal bacteria beneficial or harmful?

Stasis and autointoxication

Two theories, put forward by a number of scientists, favoured the idea of the intestinal bacteria being harmful.

The first theory was known as 'stasis': that slow movement of the faeces through the bowel was undesirable. There already existed a longstanding belief that the contents of the colon were potentially harmful, an idea that could be traced back to Ancient Egyptian and Greek civilisations.

Belief in stasis was very prevalent in the nineteenth century and was reflected in the use of 'intestinal lavage', a form of enema provided at health spas in Britain and Europe. In the U.S.A. they were described as 'colon laundries'.[7]

A similar theory stated that the putrefactive bacteria in the colon were producing poisons (toxins), which entered the body and caused disease. This second theory was known as 'autointoxication'.

The two theories, stasis and autointoxication, encouraged the use of purgatives for 'purification'. For instance, if a patient was feeling listless, a laxative or enema might be prescribed. It was thought that slowness of the bowels was allowing toxins to build up and be absorbed into the body, causing the listlessness.

Although there was little evidence to support the theory of autointoxication, it was nevertheless adopted by an eminent English surgeon, Sir W. Arbuthnot Lane. In the early part of the twentieth century, he undertook a range of surgical operations to alter the position of the intestines, theoretically to increase the flow of contents, with a view to treating a wide range of generalised symptoms.

Increasingly, the colon was seen as an obsolete and potentially dangerous part of the body. Eventually, Lane introduced the surgical removal of the colon as a cure for 'autointoxication diseases'. This procedure was carried out on an estimated 1,000 patients.

Nobel Prize winner condemns the colon

The negative view of the colon and its contents was shared by a key figure in the history of probiotics, Elie Metchnikoff a Russian zoologist. Metchnikoff gained eminence through his work in discovering phagocytes (cells that attack bacteria), for which he was awarded the Nobel Prize.

While working at the Pasteur Institute in Paris at the turn of the twentieth century, Metchnikoff declared his support for the autointoxication theory. In one of his books he described the large intestine as "the reservoir of the waste of the digestive processes, and the waste stagnates long enough to putrefy. The products of putrefaction are harmful".[8]

For a while he was attracted by the idea of Lane's extreme surgical method of dealing with the colon, but eventually rejected it. Instead, Metchnikoff concluded that the bacterial population of the intestines could be improved by adding beneficial bacteria.

Metchnikoff's adoption of the idea of beneficial bacteria arose from his enquiries into how old age could be delayed and life prolonged.

Metchnikoff and Bulgarian peasants

In his wide-ranging enquiries Metchnikoff became interested in a population of mountain peasants in Bulgaria who were known for their longevity. He thought that the fermented milk they drank had a role to play in their long life. Metchnikoff reckoned that by consuming soured milk products the human microflora could be changed and improved.

He found a bacterium in the peasants' milk, and named it *Bacillus bulgaricus*. Metchnikoff argued that the lactic acid produced by the bacterium reduced the harmful effects of other micro-organisms.

Because of inadequate records, it is not certain which bacterium Metchnikoff identified. It may have been *Lactobacillus delbrueckii* subsp. *bulgaricus*, a strain of bacteria commonly used today as a starter culture for yoghurts.

The fashion for fermented milk products

As a consequence of scientific legitimacy given by Metchnikoff's theory, it became fashionable in the early part of the twentieth century in Europe to consume fermented milk products.

One observer commented on the enthusiasm in Britain. "For several months one heard of nothing but the Bulgarian bacillus. The bacillus shared with Lloyd George's budget the honor of monopolizing the conversation at the dinner tables of the great. He [the bacillus] dominated Belgravia, frolicked in Fulham, and bestrode Birmingham and the whole of the British Isles".[9] In his history of bacteriologists, Paul de Kruif wrote in 1926, "The Bulgarian bacillus became a rage, companies were formed, and the directors grew rich off selling these silly bacilli".[10]

It is understandable why fermented milks should have become popular. There was the long-standing belief that the contents of the lower intestines were undesirable, which is hardly surprising as solid waste is passed out of the body and may be foul smelling. This belief was supported by leading scientists and medics of the time.

There was also the romantic idea that rural peasants lived longer lives because of something they ate, and that this food could be brought to urban areas. Thirdly, there was the fear that if people did not do something to improve their bowels, their colons might be surgically removed.

The theories fall apart

The popularity of fermented milk in the early part of the twentieth century faded because of several developments.

First, a range of scientific experiments showed that the autointoxication theory was incorrect. Toxins produced in the colon were not responsible for the illnesses that Lane and others medics claimed.

Secondly, Metchnikoff died in 1916 at the age of 71. In those days this was a good age, but as Metchnikoff had spent his last fifteen years consuming large quantities of sour milk with the Bulgarian bacillus, and many people believed this would extend his life substantially, his death further weakened support for his theories.

Following Metchnikoff's death, Leo F. Rettger at Yale University investigated the two bacteria used in yoghurt production (*L. bulgaricus* and *Streptococcus thermophilus*). He found that most were killed off by stomach acid and intestinal bile salts. He also found that *L. bulgaricus* did not colonise the gut and was therefore a transient bacterium, less likely to affect the intestines.[11]

Vitamins and minerals were discovered and their importance to health established. Vitamins were actively investigated and identified in the 1920s, particularly at the Lister Institute in London. Scientific opinion assumed that the perceived benefits from fermented milks were the result of vitamins and minerals, rather than lactic acid bacteria.

And finally, medical interest in beneficial bacteria waned further with the development of antibiotics, following the discovery of penicillin by Alexander Fleming in 1928. The focus shifted to the use of antibiotics in controlling infectious diseases, through the inhibition and killing of bacteria. There seemed to be no need for the ingestion of beneficial bacteria when antibiotics could destroy the harmful ones.

As a result of these developments, ideas that the large intestine was unnecessary and that its contents were harmful, together with the notion that fermented milks could help prolong life, lost support among physicians.

The argument about whether the huge numbers of bacteria in the colon were 'good' or 'bad' had swung from definitely harmful to neither particularly 'bad' nor 'good'.

The surgeon Sir W. Arbuthnot Lane was still highly thought of for his skilled and innovative techniques, and Metchnikoff was still highly regarded for his work on the immune system. But both were viewed as having erred in the later stages of their careers by supporting the autointoxication theory.

With the decline in support from the medical profession, public interest in fermented drinks also fell away.

Was Metchnikoff really wrong?

By the end of the twentieth century, Metchnikoff's reputation had been enhanced, because:

- toxins produced by putrefactive bacteria in slow-moving stools are now associated with cancer of the colon;
- the normal microflora has been shown, on balance, to be slightly more harmful than beneficial;[12]
- evidence is accumulating for the use of probiotic bacteria for prevention and treatment of disease (for example, infectious diarrhoea);
- the health value of fermented milks, through the by-products of fermentation, is being recognised. (The Bulgarian peasants probably did benefit from consuming fermented milk, even if it was unlikely to have been a major factor in their longevity.)

Even in the earlier part of the twentieth century, interest in fermented milks among the general public did not die out completely. There was a continuing demand for these milks as there was something about them that people found beneficial. The continuing demand made it feasible for companies to pursue commercial production.

Early commercial products

In 1919 the Danone company was formed in Barcelona, Spain. Today this company is a major producer of 'functional foods', that is, foods that have health benefits in addition to normal nutrition.[13] In Europe, Danone produces two major probiotic products: Actimel®, a fermented milk drink, and Bio Activia® yoghurt. Both contain probiotic bacteria (a lactobacillus and a bifidobacterium, respectively).

In the United States, the Yale scientist Leo F. Rettger switched his attention away from *L. bulgaricus* towards other lactic-acid bacteria, especially *Lactobacillus acidophilus*. He found that various preparations using this bacterium helped to alleviate constipation and to improve diarrhoea.[14] Rettger's work helped the development of commercial products in the U.S.A., such as acidophilus milk (unfermented milk with *L. acidophilus* added).

In Japan in 1930, Dr Minoru Shirota, a microbiologist, identified a lactic acid bacterium resistant to stomach acid, later named *L. casei* Shirota. By 1935 his company had produced a milk drink with the name Yakult (Esperanto for yoghurt). This subsequently proved very popular in Japan and is today delivered to workplaces by travelling salespeople known as Yakult Ladies, of whom there are currently more than 50,000. The Yakult company produces many other items, including skin products. It has also expanded, more recently, to Europe and North America.

Although for most of last century a health product popular in Japan was not of much interest to people in the rest of the world,[15] now both yoghurts and probiotic milk products are so popular there is a wide choice in most supermarkets in the Western world. Something changed to make them popular.

The cause of stomach ulcers

One factor in the change in public attitudes to the health-giving characteristics of beneficial bacteria may have been a further change of opinion in the medical profession about the importance of bacteria in the intestines.

It used to be thought that stomach ulcers were caused by excessive stress, often related to the demands of work. The prevalent theory was that a stressed individual produced more stomach acid than was necessary to digest food and that this excess acid harmed the lining of the stomach and the duodenum (first part of the small intestine).

In 1982, however, two Australian researchers, Barry Marshall and Robin Warren, put forward a theory that stomach ulcers were caused by a spiral-shaped bacterium named *Helicobacter pylori*. This theory was so contrary to conventional wisdom that a major debate ensued. Criticism of the Australians was fierce. As they were so sure that their theory was correct, and because they wanted to win over the doubters, Marshall and another colleague infected themselves with *H. pylori*. Both men developed gastritis (inflammation of the stomach and duodenum).

They recovered from the gastritis once they took antibiotics, which strengthened the argument that a bacterium was the cause of gastric ulcers.

Other researchers also showed that antibiotics healed ulcers and prevented recurrence in 90 per cent of cases. The U.S. Government-funded National Institutes of Health monitored the research closely and in 1994 concluded that *H. pylori* "plays a significant role in the development of ulcers".

The acceptance by the scientific establishment of this explanation had a profound effect on medical thought, and has been described as "one of the most chastening lessons in gastroenterology this century, and has heightened awareness of the role of bacteria in the gut".[16]

If bacteria were the key to one particular gastrointestinal disease, they might be important to others. It thus followed that there was fresh interest in bacteria as a possible cause of Ulcerative Colitis and Crohn's Disease.

In parallel with the medical profession, the veterinary profession was also changing its attitude towards gut bacteria.

Antibiotics for animals

During the Second World War, the supply of food to the U.K. by sea had been greatly disrupted. The British Government of the time was very conscious of this vulnerability and, after the war, encouraged the more efficient production of food within Britain to enhance self-sufficiency.

Intensive meat production methods were adopted. This meant keeping chickens, pigs and other animals in large buildings crowded together. Although this method was more efficient in producing meat, it also increased the risk of spreading infectious diseases.

The usual way of treating bacterial diseases is to provide antibiotics. With intensively reared animals living close together, however, bacterial disease could easily be passed to other animals before the antibiotic worked. Therefore it became the practice, once one animal had become infected, to give antibiotics to all animals living in one barn together, by adding the drugs to water or food.

Despite the mass use of antibiotics, substantial harm could still be done to the animals before the infectious disease was brought under control.

Instead of relying on mass treatment, farmers began to use antibiotics before any infection had occurred. Thus, from the 1950s onwards, the use of antibiotics grew rapidly as farmers used them

2: The History of Probiotics

as prophylactics (for prevention).

Then something surprising happened. The low-level use of antibiotics to prevent disease led to animals putting on weight (3 to 11 per cent more, depending on the species of animal). The reason was not clear, although it was suspected that among the bacterial flora killed by the antibiotics there was one or more species that was holding back the animals' growth.

Naturally, farmers were pleased with the increased income resulting from selling animals of heavier weight. Feed companies started adding antibiotics to animal food and described them as 'growth promoters'.

Antibiotic-resistant bacteria

The problem with the continual use of antibiotics is that while many harmful bacteria are killed or inhibited, some will survive, and these are more likely to be ones that are resistant to the anti-bacterial effects of the antibiotics. These resistant bacteria may increase in numbers because the competing bacteria in the microflora are weakened or eliminated (because antibiotics tend to kill 'good' and 'bad' bacteria alike).

Thus, with the use of antibiotics as prophylactics and growth promoters, there was a rise in the number of farmed animals containing antibiotic-resistant bacteria as part of their gut flora.

Politicians and other influential people became fearful that this resistance would spread to humans and lead to outbreaks of infectious diseases that could not be easily controlled by antibiotics.

Since their discovery and development, antibiotic drugs have had a tremendous effect in controlling infectious diseases, and as a consequence premature death, particularly in infants, has fallen dramatically. In fact, antibiotics have proved so successful it was thought by many that the war had been won against disease in humans. Therefore, it was an alarming idea that antibiotics might have adverse effects through their over-use in modern farming.

The Swann Committee

In the late 1960s, the British Government set up a committee, chaired by Professor M. M. Swann, to examine the use of antibiotics in farmed animals. Reporting in 1969, the Swann committee concluded that "the administration of antibiotics to farm livestock, particularly at sub-therapeutic levels, poses certain hazards to human and animal health". They recommended that antibiotics used in treating human disease should not be used as growth promoters in farmed animals.

The committee did not recommend a complete ban on all antibiotics as growth promoters because of a fear that some farmers might be pushed into bankruptcy. Also, use of any antibiotics in animals for prophylactic purposes was still allowed.

Legislation was passed in line with the Swann recommendations, but, as the dividing line between growth promotion and mass prophylaxis is not altogether clear, the reduction in the use of 'human' antibiotics was not as great as had been hoped. It has been estimated that about one half (by volume) of all antibiotics used in the UK is for non-human use, which demonstrates the continuing large-scale use of antibiotics by farmers. Consequently, the debate about antibiotic-resistance transferring from animals to humans is still continuing.

A world-wide concern

This continuing concern was reflected in a conference held in 1994 by the World Health Organisation (WHO) to discuss resistance to antibiotics. The WHO Scientific Working Group stated that the incidence of resistance "has increased at an alarming rate in recent years and is expected to increase at a similar or even greater rate in the future as antimicrobial agents continue to lose their effectiveness".[17]

In addition to recommending a reduction in the use of antibiotics, the WHO Group also suggested the use of 'bacterial interference', an alternative phrase for probiotics.

Probiotics for animals

It was for the farming industry that probiotics, as separate products rather than as part of fermented drinks, were first developed commercially.

From the early 1970s in the U.K., the ban on the use of certain antibiotics as growth promoters for farmed animals had the effect of making some farmers more open to alternatives for keeping their intensively farmed animals healthy.

There was another factor that made farmers receptive to the

concept of probiotics: the regular use of antibiotics had the undesirable consequence of increasing the incidence of diarrhoea amongst the animals, thus weakening them.

Antibiotics were killing the normal benign and beneficial gut bacteria. In the resulting 'vacuum' other more harmful bacteria had the chance of becoming established in the intestines and causing diarrhoea.

Why was it thought that probiotics might be helpful for farmed animals? The only form of probiotic at that time was fermented milk, and it was not obvious, for example, that yoghurt should be fed to chickens.

Incubator-hatched chickens are much more susceptible to salmonella infection than free-range chickens. A reasonable explanation for this is that because the incubator-hatched chickens hatch and grow in a clean environment, they do not acquire the normal gut flora from their mother. Reconstituting that flora might help resistance to infection.

In 1973, two Finnish veterinarians extracted samples of the intestinal contents of healthy chickens and transferred the samples into the throats of newly hatched chicks, which then passed into their intestines. Resistance to harmful salmonella bacteria was greater in the treated chicks than in those chicks that did not receive any transferred gut contents.[18]

This study strengthened the belief that a well-balanced gut microflora was an important factor in animal health, and led to a search to identify which bacteria in the normal microflora were important for providing protection against disease.

Feed company research

Feed companies undertook many tests to find out which microbes benefited what animals. The identification of useful species and strains for animal probiotics came mostly through private research. Little of that research has been published in peer-reviewed journals, so the information needed to judge the reliability of the research is often missing.

One reviewer of research into probiotics on chickens commented that many experiments were reported as abstracts of oral communications presented at meetings and that "some of the interpretation of results is obviously overly optimistic".[19]

The weakness of studies into probiotics for animals did not discourage farmers. In their experience, these beneficial bacteria reduced the incidence of diarrhoea and other infections in their animals. Thus demand for these products grew.

Feed companies and others related to farming developed a wide range of products. As many as twenty-six different species of bacteria and three fungi have been used in animal probiotic products.[20]

Probiotics become fashionable again

The fact that farmers were confident about the use of probiotics in farm animals did not mean that probiotic products would automatically be developed for humans. Other factors were at work.

In the last decade of the twentieth century, interest in probiotics among the general public steadily increased. Probiotic food products, mostly milk-based, started to appear in supermarkets, and probiotic supplements appeared in health-food stores.

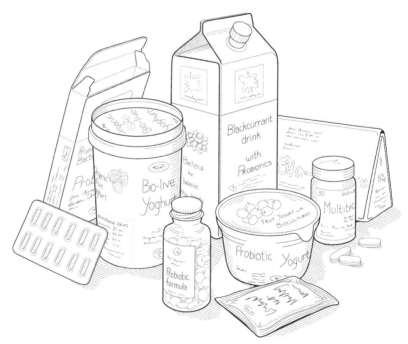

Fig 4. Different types of probiotic products

2: The History of Probiotics

There are probably three main explanations for this. First, whilst the incidence of premature death from disease declined rapidly during the twentieth century, and human health in general has improved, digestive disorders continue to be common and troublesome.

Secondly, there has been a growing public concern about the increased and sometimes excessive use of pharmaceutical products, including antibiotics, often with associated side effects.

Thirdly, the concept of wholistic health, in which overall body systems are improved, rather than targeting a specific disease, has grown in popularity.

Within this context, the general public has been receptive to the idea of improving the intestines and the immune system by adding 'friendly bacteria'. However, it is also fair to say that understanding of how probiotics work is poor, and is often little more than a feeling that these products are 'good for you'.

Having said that, the beginning of the twenty-first century has probably seen an end to the ridiculing of Metchnikoff's ideas on beneficial bacteria, which he first proposed one hundred years ago. Now, the lay public and medics are receptive to the idea of probiotics, both in aiding good health and treating illness.

Chapter summary

- A probiotic is "A live microbial feed supplement which beneficially affects the host animal by improving its intestinal microbial balance".[2]

- Bacterial fermentation of food and drink, to improve flavour and act as a preservative, has been in evidence for thousands of years.

- Scientists began to learn about bacteria from the mid-nineteenth century onwards.

- There has been an ongoing debate about whether bacteria in the colon are good or bad.

- Metchnikoff was the first scientist to propose that health can be improved by adding lactic acid bacteria to the diet, through fermented milks.

- The enthusiasm for beneficial bacteria in the early part of the twentieth century soon faded because of three main developments.

- The theories of stasis and autointoxication were discredited, due to exaggerated claims and lack of supportive scientific evidence; the discovery of vitamins provided an alternative explanation (to lactic acid bacteria) for the apparent health benefits of fermented milks; and the development of antibiotics switched attention from the merits of beneficial bacteria to the merits of destroying bacteria.

- Towards the end of the twentieth century new information showed that Metchnikoff was essentially correct in his assessment that:
  - some bacteria in the colon produce harmful toxins;
  - lactic acid bacteria have health benefits; and
  - fermented milks are nutritious.

- The demand for fermented drinks by the general public throughout the twentieth century meant that companies such as Danone and Yakult were able to grow and continue their research.

- The discovery that a bacterium, *H. pylori,* was a cause of stomach and duodenal ulcers, increased medical interest in bacteria as a possible cause of other intestinal conditions, including IBD.

- The use of antibiotics in intensively reared farm animals increased greatly, to treat and prevent bacterial infections and improve the growth of animals.

- The use of antibiotics led to an increase in antibiotic resistant bacteria in animals.

- In some countries, restrictions on the use of antibiotics in animals led farmers to develop an interest in probiotics, as an alternative way of controlling diarrhoea and infectious diseases.

- The knowledge gained by developing a range of probiotics for animals formed the basis for developing probiotics for humans.

- Interest in probiotic products among the general public grew substantially in the last decade of the twentieth century.

3. IBD, Bacteria & Inflammation

"For the first few years of having colitis of the rectum, I had several remission periods. But at the end of 2000 and during the greater part of 2001, I suffered mucus and bleeding. After taking various prescribed medicines in 2002 there was an improvement. However, after taking a probiotic milk drink for a month my situation improved dramatically. I am now practically 'normal' and my consultant told me to keep taking the probiotic drink and come back to see him in a year."

Why should probiotics, which have become increasingly popular in recent years, have any effect on IBD? What is it about Crohn's and UC that might make these diseases of the gut respond to beneficial bacteria?

To help answer these two questions, it is first necessary to consider the relationship between IBD, bacteria and inflammation.

Inflammatory Bowel Disease (IBD)

IBD is a general term for two related conditions: Ulcerative Colitis and Crohn's Disease. They are chronic (on-going) conditions that are much more common in developed countries of the world, affecting as many as one in 500 of the population. The teen and young-adult years are often the time when these diseases start; and currently there is no cure (other than, for UC, the surgical removal of the colon).

The symptoms of IBD include severe and persistent diarrhoea (sometimes with blood and mucus), tiredness, pain, loss of weight and sometimes constipation. There may be non-intestinal problems such as arthritis and inflammation of the eyes. Treatment usually involves anti-inflammatory and immuno-suppressive drugs, and these may cause unpleasant side effects.

The diseases fluctuate unpredictably, with 'flare-ups' and periods of remission. Some people are rarely troubled by their IBD, while others are almost permanently distressed and require surgery to remove part of their intestine.

UC affects only the colon (large intestine) and/or the rectum, while Crohn's may occur anywhere in the digestive tract from the mouth to the anus. It is worth noting that the most common places of inflammation in IBD are at the terminal ileum (the very end of the small intestine) and in the colon.

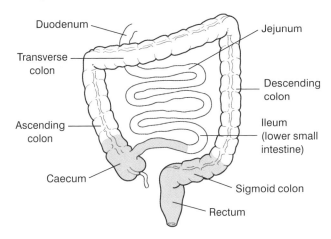

Fig 5. Parts of the intestine most commonly affected by IBD

What are bacteria?

Bacteria are tiny single-cell creatures that can only be viewed through a microscope. While the great majority of bacteria live outside the human body (in soil, plants, water and air), there are some bacteria that live inside animals, including humans.

There are so many bacteria living inside us that it has been calculated that they outnumber human cells by up to 10 to one.[1]

Bacteria are found in the mouth, all through the intestine and in the vagina. The great majority (85 per cent) are found in the colon. The other area where there is a particularly large concentration of bacteria is the ileum (the last part of the small intestine).

The largest concentrations of bacteria are, therefore, found in the parts of the intestine most frequently affected by IBD.

3: IBD, Bacteria & Inflammation

The number of bacteria

Bacteria are counted as numbers of cfu, short for 'colony forming units'; that is, the number alive and in a state to multiply and form a group. The average number of bacteria in different parts of the digestive tract is listed below:

- in the stomach, less than 1,000 cfu (per millilitre of gut contents);
- the duodenum, about 1,000–10,000 cfu/ml;
- the jejunum (main part of small intestine), up to 100,000 cfu/ml;
- the ileum, up to 100 million cfu/ml;
- the colon, 10 billion–1 trillion cfu per gram of contents.[2]

The numbers of bacteria increase along the small intestine, from the duodenum to the ileum. In the colon, the numbers get even larger. In fact, the numbers of bacteria in the colon are about 100 million times greater than in the stomach.

Another way of looking at the huge numbers involved is to try to imagine how many bacteria there are in one gram of the contents of the colon.

It has been calculated that the number is, on average, 150 times greater than the total number of human beings living on planet earth.[3]

Why not remove all bacteria in the human gut?

As bacteria appear to be associated with IBD, perhaps the best solution would be to remove the bacteria and the IBD might stop. This idea is given weight by research which shows that mice with colitis will get better if all intestinal bacteria are removed through the use of antibiotics.[4]

There are two reasons why a bacteria-free gut is not a solution.

First, the intestines would not remain free from bacteria for long. Millions upon millions of bacteria enter the body every day (chiefly through the nose and mouth) and some of them will inevitably colonise the intestines. Taking antibiotics continuously would keep them at bay, but long-term use of antibiotics carries the risk of encouraging antibiotic-resistant bacteria; if dominant, these bacteria may cause further disease, which might be difficult to treat.

The second reason why a bacteria-free gut is not a solution to IBD

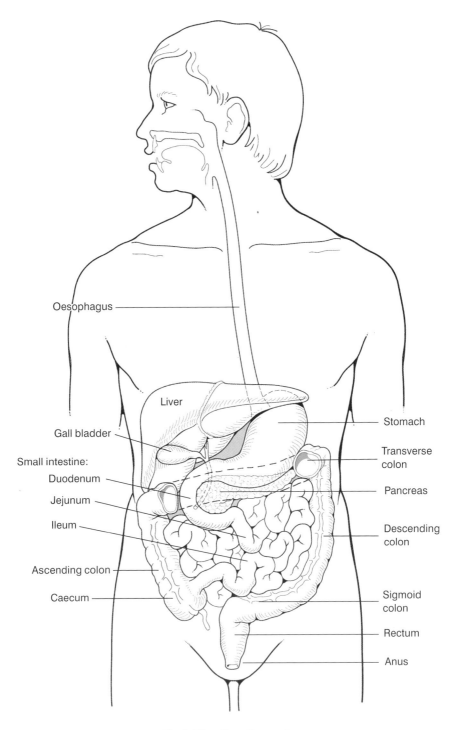

Fig 6. The digestive system

is that the normal gut bacteria, in addition to being associated with IBD, also have some desirable effects. The microflora (all the tiny organisms in the gut) benefit the body in ways that are only now being discovered; for example, improved immune system, vitamin and nutrient production, and a barrier against harmful infections.

The cause of IBD

Although most gut bacteria are found in the parts of the intestine most commonly affected by IBD inflammation, this does not prove that bacteria cause IBD. An association is not proof of a causal relationship.

At present, the cause of IBD is not known. The favoured scientific theory, however, points to bacterial involvement.

The theory is that a pathogen (a tiny harmful agent), possibly a bacterium, reaches the intestine in large numbers and triggers the immune system (part of the body's defences). Inflammation results from the response made by the immune system, but instead of stopping when the pathogen has been defeated, the inflammation carries on as though there were dangerous invaders still present.

It is thought that the immune system continues the inflammation by mistakenly reacting to the normal gut microflora.

Why doesn't everyone develop IBD?

If everyone has bacteria in their intestine and we all come in contact with a huge range of pathogens that might trigger the disease, why doesn't everyone develop IBD?

IBD is not contagious. If there is a pathogen that initiates Crohn's or UC, the disease will not start just because the pathogen is present. Other factors, either environmental (for example, lifestyle, where you live) or genetic, must be present.

A gene associated with Crohn's Disease has already been identified. Other genes, for both UC and for Crohn's, are expected to be identified in the future.

It is also clear that IBD is not caused solely by a genetic variation. In identical twins there have been instances of one twin having IBD and the other not, even though they share exactly the same genes.

Possible triggers of IBD

If the theory set out above is correct, which microbe (microscopic organism) initiates inflammation? Several different microbes have been considered as possible triggers:

- *Mycobacterium paratuberculosis*; a microbe common in some cattle populations which causes disease. A minority of scientists believe that its presence in the milk supply, in some countries, is a factor in causing Crohn's Disease.

- The measles virus; in particular, its use in a weakened form together with two other viruses in the MMR (measles, mumps, rubella) vaccine administered to children in the U.K. and other countries.

- A helicobacter bacterium; since the role of *H. pylori* in stomach and duodenal ulcers was discovered.

- Members of the normal human microflora; for example, *Bacteroides vulgatis, Enterococcus faecalis, Escherichia coli, Desulfovibrio desulfuricans.*

Nevertheless, in an expert review, John Cummings and George Macfarlane concluded that, "no single pathogen or group of organisms that determine IBD is presently accepted".[5]

Mucosal permeability

Whether the trigger that initiates IBD is an external microbe, or something that is part of the normal microflora, initial inflammation is likely to be set off by a pathogen entering through the mucosa (mucus-lined inner gut wall).

The epithelial cells of the mucosa let digested nutrients into the blood stream and keep out harmful agents. But this arrangement may not work well in people who have IBD. Microbes may pass through the intestinal wall too easily. This increased mucosal permeability is known as 'leaky gut'.

If bacteria in the colon and ileum are likely to be a factor in IBD, why doesn't it develop as soon as the intestinal bacteria have established themselves in early childhood?

We don't know. It may be that an unusual pathogen triggers the inflammation. Perhaps the person has to have a weak immune system that reacts incorrectly to the microbial trigger. Or possibly a particular genetic response may occur only when a combination of factors happen at the same time.

Probiotic relief

The theory behind probiotic use for IBD is that, by changing the types of bacteria in the colon and ileum, the immune system will stop reacting incorrectly, the inflammation will cease and the intestines will recover.

How might probiotic bacteria accomplish this? They might:

- attach themselves to the surface of the intestinal wall, increase in numbers and make it more difficult for harmful bacteria to become established;
- compete for nutrients more successfully than less desirable bacteria;
- make the intestines more acidic, which harmful bacteria do not tolerate;
- produce bacteriocides (chemicals that discourage or kill other bacteria);
- affect the immune system so that it acts correctly.

Understanding inflammation

To understand better how probiotics may work for IBD, let us first understand what inflammation involves.

Inflammation is an important part of the immune system, which in turn is part of the body's defences. Inflammation is a process whereby there is an increase in the supply of blood to an infected area. The extra blood contains white blood cells that attack the invading harmful agents.

The extra blood flooding into the affected tissues makes the area red and swollen. The pressure of the extra blood in the tissues causes tenderness. If the inflammation is on the skin it feels hot, as the blood is closer than usual to the surface.

For example, if you have a splinter in one of your fingers, the surrounding area becomes inflamed; the tissue becomes red, swollen, hot and tender. Also, some of its function, that is, its ability to do its job, may be lost.

Pain

If UC and Crohn's are inflammatory diseases, why doesn't the intestine feel tender and painful all the time, like an inflamed gum or finger? The reason is that the lining of the intestine has almost no pain-sensing cells and therefore little feeling. This is why a person with IBD can have a stoma, in which an end of the intestine is brought to the surface of the abdomen, and experience little discomfort when a bag is attached (for collecting excreted bodily waste).

The muscles that surround the intestine can, however, sense pain. These muscles can be affected in Crohn's Disease, as the inflammation is usually present through the whole of the wall of the intestine, rather than just in the lining as is the case with UC. Therefore, when the gut muscles strain to force food down the intestines, this can lead to pain for those with Crohn's. This is why pain is a more common symptom in Crohn's than in UC.

Pain in UC is usually felt only in the rectum as this is the one part of the intestine where the lining does have feeling.

Heat

Heat is felt on inflamed skin, because the temperature of the surrounding skin is cooler than the extra blood that has temporarily been diverted towards the surface. Inflammation inside the body does not feel hot, however, as the intestine is the same temperature as the blood in the body. Thus, although the intestinal inflammation of IBD is similar to inflammation elsewhere in the body, involving a reddening and swelling of the tissues, tenderness and heat are not normally felt.

Loss of function

If you have a wound on your hand, inflammation will follow and may be so severe that it will not be possible to hold things properly. The hand will have lost part of its function. Similarly, if you have arthritis of the knee, the joint may be so inflamed that you cannot move your knee fully and so will have walking restrictions.

If the bowel is inflamed, the ability of the body to absorb nutrients and water may be impaired and control of bowel movements may also be reduced. Some function may therefore be lost because of inflammation.

The battlefield

If inflammation is part of the defence against harmful invaders, why does it have certain negative consequences, such as loss of function?

Inflammation can be viewed as the site of a battle between invading pathogens and the defending immune cells. In any battle, there are casualties on both sides and the battlefield becomes scarred.

This is what happens with IBD. A battle takes place within the tissues of the intestine and they become scarred. It is frustrating that the 'invading enemy' is not known, and that the battle (inflammation) is maintained because the body has become confused as to whom the enemy is.

What exactly happens when tissue becomes inflamed? To understand this, you need to have a basic understanding of the body's defence systems, particularly the immune system.

The body's defence systems

The human body defends itself from attacking microbes by three main methods:

- physical barriers
- the innate immune system
- the adaptive immune system

The physical barriers

The physical barriers stop the great majority of harmful organisms from entering the body and becoming established. The barriers are:

- skin
- mucus (a sticky substance that lines the lungs, nose, intestine and vagina)
- gastric acid (that kills the great majority of microbes that enter the stomach)
- peristalsis (muscle contractions of the intestines that keep food moving and make it difficult for bacteria to become established).[6]

The innate immune system

The innate immune system is a quick acting set of white blood cells, proteins and chemicals that are stimulated into action when microbes enter the bloodstream. Together, they destroy the most common invaders. The father of probiotics, Elie Metchnikoff, gained his Nobel Prize by discovering phagocytes, one type of these white blood cells.

Chemicals released by white blood cells cause inflammation. The chemicals have a funnel-like effect in the area under attack, making it easier for blood to get in and more difficult for it to get out. This is achieved through changing the spaces between cells. The increased amount of blood in the inflamed tissue enables more of the defending white blood cells to be present and increases the chances that they will outnumber and defeat the harmful invading microbes.

When the inflammatory battle takes place in the gut wall, the damaged tissues will bleed, more mucus will be produced to flush away the microbes, and pus (dead white blood cells) may be produced. That is why blood, mucus and pus are sometimes found in the stools of people with IBD.

The adaptive immune system

The adaptive immune system can deal with all invading microbes. It takes longer to get going than the innate system and involves the production of antibodies, which are proteins that attach themselves to the invading microbes. Once the antibodies are attached to the pathogens it is easier for the phagocytes to destroy the invaders.

The type of white blood cells that produce antibodies are called B cells. They find the invaders most easily in the lymph system, which is a set of vessels that exist parallel with and connected to the blood vessels.

The B cells are extraordinary, because they can produce millions of different types of antibodies, each one specific to a particular invader.[7]

For a fuller description of the body's defence systems, see Appendix 1.

The immune system and IBD

The immune system is very complicated. There are many different elements that, to a greater or lesser extent, are interrelated.

Because of the very complicated chemical processes involved when the human immune system is active, the action of the immune system in IBD is still not fully understood.

It should not be surprising that our immune systems are complicated; if all of the different layers of the defence failed, then we would die. As a consequence, however, if the system goes partly wrong, as with IBD, it is not particularly straightforward to fix. Researchers are, however, steadily getter a better picture of the different elements involved.

3: IBD, Bacteria & Inflammation

Mucosal immune system

Some researchers examine the physical barriers (for example, the mucus lining the intestine). Others examine the 'transport routes' of blood and lymph that are relevant to non-intestinal symptoms of IBD (for instance, arthritis, inflammation of the eyes).

The vital area for researching the core IBD symptoms (diarrhoea and weakness) is, however, the collection of immune cells and chemicals associated with the gut wall and lining, known as the 'mucosal immune system'. It has been discovered that a great many immune processes are interconnected just within the mucosa (inner gut wall).

The mucosal immune system acts subtly because it has to differentiate between harmful and beneficial microscopic particles passing through the intestine wall into the bloodstream. It has to stimulate attacks on pathogenic micro-organisms entering the blood, and at the same time has to downplay reaction to tiny digested food particles that need to be absorbed into the body.[8]

It is known that certain types of white blood cells play a role in IBD. They are T-helper cells that can move into the intestine. One type of T-helper cells (Th1) produce pro-inflammatory proteins while another (Th2) produce anti-inflammatory proteins. In people with IBD, the Th1 cells seem to be overactive, while the Th2 cells appear to respond abnormally.[9]

Researchers are looking at ways in which the T-helper cells can be affected to bring IBD inflammation to an end.

Treatments for IBD

Current treatment for IBD focuses on breaking the cycle of continuing inflammation. Drugs such as corticosteroids are used to suppress the immune response.

A new wave of drugs involves targeting a particular element in the immune response. The first of such drugs is infliximab, an antibody against a pro-inflammatory protein (TNF-alpha).

Future treatment may involve altering the faulty genes that are thought to be a factor in IBD.

Gut bacteria are also involved in treatment. Antibiotics can often help improve Crohn's, but also they may kill or weaken a large part of the normal microflora.

Probiotics fit within this picture of treatments. Rather than disturb the microflora, as do antibiotics, probiotics may be able to work with the microflora to break the cycle of continuing inflammation, and so bring relief to those distressed by IBD.

Chapter summary

- IBD is a chronic (on-going) inflammation of the intestine. Symptoms include diarrhoea, tiredness, pain and loss of weight, and may involve inflammation of other parts of the body.

- Huge numbers of bacteria live in our intestines, especially in the terminal ileum (the very end of the small intestine) and the colon.

- IBD is usually found in the parts of the intestine where there are most bacteria, but it is not practical (or necessarily desirable) to remove the bacterial flora from the intestine.

- Although the cause of IBD is not yet known, a current popular theory is that a pathogen triggers the immune system. The inflammation fails to stop when the pathogen is defeated, and continues to be stimulated incorrectly by the normal gut bacteria.

- Immune system malfunction is thought to be affected by genes and environmental factors. IBD is not contagious.

- There is no agreement as to what particular microbes might trigger the inflammation or even if there is an external trigger.

- Permeability of the gut wall may be a factor in IBD.

- Probiotics are thought to work by several methods (attachment to the gut wall, competing for nutrients, making the content of the intestine more acidic, producing anti-bacterial chemicals and stimulating the immune system), to stop or reduce the continuing inflammation.

- Inflammation is part of the body's process of defending itself from invading pathogens. It involves letting blood flood into an infected area to enable the white blood cells to do battle with the invading microbes.

- Inflammation temporarily reduces the ability of the inflamed part of the body to function properly. Inflamed intestine is less able to absorb salts and water, and so diarrhoea develops.

- The body's defence system consists of physical barriers, and the innate and adaptive immune systems.
- · Researchers into IBD are devoting much attention to the mucosal immune system which has an important role in the development and continuation of UC and Crohn's.
- Current drug treatments for IBD suppress the immune system, or reduce the amount of inflammatory chemicals (for example, TNF-alpha). Future treatment may involve altering faulty genes, and/or manipulating the gut bacteria with antibiotics and probiotics.

4. Probiotics for IBD: Evidence for benefits

"My Crohn's was diagnosed nine years ago following bowel obstruction. Over the years I have had fairly regular acute episodes and two operations. I also had to give up my career as a Senior Nurse. For the past six months I have been taking one probiotic milk drink in the morning, a yoghurt at lunch, and another drink before bed. My general health and quality of life has increased tenfold, and I have been able to take up employment again in a responsible position."

A malfunction of the immune system is likely to be involved in the cause and continuance of IBD. Although the immune system is complex, making it difficult to resolve UC and Crohn's, it may be possible to find scientific evidence for the use of probiotics.

Eight substantial reviews on the subject of probiotics and IBD were published at the turn of the twenty-first century in journals or specialist books.[1-8]

What have these experts said about probiotics and IBD?

Evidence for the importance of bacteria

Several general points were made. Michael Schultz and Balfour Sartor stated that the "luminal bacterial flora plays a major role in initiation and perpetuation of chronic inflammatory bowel disease".[1] (Luminal refers to the lumen, the space within the intestinal tube).

William Faubion and William Sandborn identified the terminal ileum, the caecum (beginning of the colon), and the rectum as areas of relatively slow movement of the bowel contents (faeces), "providing prolonged mucosal contact with luminal contents". Those areas are particularly common places for inflammation in IBD.[2]

Cummings and Macfarlane observed that the "inflammatory response seen in the mucosa of both Crohn's disease and ulcerative colitis closely mimics known bacterial infections of the gut".[3]

Clinical experience

Several reviewers pointed to clinical experience of reducing Crohn's Disease activity through the use of antibiotics. Antibiotics kill bacteria, so the evidence of a connection between bacteria and Crohn's is strengthened.[3,4,5,8] Very few studies have found that antibiotics reduce UC.[9] Cummings and Macfarlane concluded, however, that this does not mean bacteria are not involved in Ulcerative Colitis, as "only a very limited range of antibiotics has been tried....and few combinations have been used".[3]

Clinical experience has also shown that Crohn's activity diminishes with 'diversion of the faecal stream', which may occur when a stoma is formed for a temporary period as part of intestinal surgery. The faeces pass through the stoma rather than passing through the colon and rectum. Surgeons and physicians have noted that the section of intestine that is no longer having faeces pass through it (while the surgery scars heal) does not develop inflammation. But as soon as the stoma is reversed and the faecal content flows through the whole of the intestine, signs of inflammation quickly return.[10,11]

Massimo Campieri and Paolo Gionchetti reported on evidence from clinical experience with pouchitis. This is an inflammatory condition of the ileo-anal pouch, a surgeon-created alternative to the colon. If the colon has to be removed, for example when Ulcerative Colitis is too severe, a reservoir or pouch is fashioned from the ileum (end of the small intestine). The pouch is then attached to the remains of the rectum to allow passage of faecal waste from the anus. It is an alternative to having a stoma on the abdomen.

The pouch has the disadvantage that a significant minority of people develop an inflammation known as pouchitis. Campieri and Gionchetti reported that pouchitis "appears to be associated with high concentrations of bacteria".[4] This is a significant observation, because people with UC do not develop inflammation of the small intestine, but they can develop inflammation of the pouch, which is reshaped small intestine (acting as a colon). This suggests that the luminal bacteria may have a powerful inflammatory effect in susceptible individuals. Pouchitis can be treated with antibiotics, which further reinforces the significance of bacteria.

Clinical experience, gained by doctors and other health professionals in the course of treating patients, is useful as a source of information to help devise theories about IBD. It is necessary, however, to undertake experiments in order to test specific aspects of the theories. This involves tests on laboratory animals, to ensure the safety and effectiveness of a treatment before conducting studies in humans.

Animal models

Many animal models for IBD have been developed, mostly in mice or rats. Experiments exploring the role of intestinal bacteria in IBD have used mice that normally develop colitis through genetic alteration or being fed irritating substances (for example, carrageenan, an extract from seaweed). By using mice that have colitis, it is possible to undertake experiments to see under what circumstances the inflammation stops.

Various studies have shown that mice that would normally develop colitis do not do so if their intestines have no bacteria (that is, born and grown in a sterile environment, or treated with antibiotics). One study used IL10-deficient mice, which do not produce a protein that reduces inflammation; as a consequence, these mice normally develop colitis. The study showed that when these mice were without intestinal bacteria they were completely free of colitis. This group of mice were kept for six months in their germ-free state and at no point did they develop colitis.[12]

The eight reviews mentioned above referenced thirteen studies that showed that colitis-prone mice with germ-free intestines did not develop colitis. Faubion and Sandborn felt these studies provided "powerful evidence that the critical component of the fecal stream is the bacteria".[2] Summarising the relevant murine studies to date, Schultz and Sartor concluded that, "These studies indicate that normal luminal bacteria are essential to the development of chronic intestinal inflammation in genetically susceptible hosts".[1]

Bacterial differences

There is some evidence that the gut bacteria in people with IBD differ from gut bacteria in healthy people.

One investigation of people with Crohn's found significantly lower levels of bifidobacteria and lactobacilli (the two main groups from which probiotic bacteria are chosen). There were also increased numbers of *Escherichia coli* in those with active Crohn's.[13]

Another study involved 30 patients with UC (12 with active disease and 18 with inactive disease) and 30 controls (people without UC). While patients with inactive UC and controls did not have any significant differences in their colonic bacteria, those with active UC had a reduction in the numbers of lactobacilli.[14]

An important recent study reported on a detailed examination of the lining of the ileum and colon. This showed a very low concentration of bacteria in healthy subjects, and a high number in patients with IBD. Furthermore, the more severe the disease the greater the number of bacteria, and the numbers in Crohn's were higher than in UC.

A wide range of species of bacteria was found on the intestinal lining. These were the same types that constitute human microflora, but in those with IBD the proportions of bacteroides and *E. coli* were substantially greater.

Because of the more sophisticated laboratory techniques used, this latest study is the strongest evidence we have so far that the numbers of various gut bacteria are different between healthy people and those with Crohn's and UC.[15]

A summary of the evidence on bacterial differences in people with IBD is that there are fewer beneficial bacteria (lactobacilli and bifidobacteria) and more of the harmful (*E. coli*) or potentially harmful bacteria (bacteroides).[5]

Bacteroides species have been found to be particularly pathogenic in experimental models,[16] and there is evidence that some bacteroides increase gut permeability through the production of toxins.[17] It should be noted that bacteroides are the most common genus of bacteria found in the colon. Therefore, IBD seems to involve increased numbers of a sometimes harmful common bacterium rather than the increase of a rare pathogen.

How to change gut bacteria

It is not clear whether the abnormal mixtures of gut bacteria in people with IBD are part of the cause or a consequence of IBD. The difference in mixture does suggest, however, that changing the bacterial balance closer to that of healthy people might be beneficial.

One way would be through the use of antibiotics. As we saw in Chapter 2, continual use of antibiotics can have the effect of promoting resistant strains of harmful bacteria. Also, as antibiotics act powerfully against bacteria it is almost impossible to manipulate the balance of species. It is more likely that whole swathes of intestinal bacteria will be wiped out, increasing the chances of the development of other infections, including infectious diarrhoea.

The other obvious route to influence the ecology of the intestinal flora is to use probiotics. But what evidence is there for certain specific probiotic bacteria in reducing the activity of IBD?

Evidence for benefits of probiotics in IBD

Campieri and Gionchetti stated that changing the microflora through "direct supplementation with protective [probiotic] bacteria .... exerts a protective role in intestinal inflammatory disease".[4]

Several studies have shown encouraging results with probiotic therapy in experimental (animal) models of IBD. Renata Fabia and colleagues induced colitis in rats with acetic acid. Some of the rats also received *Lactobacillus reuteri* immediately after acetic acid, and colitis was prevented.[18]

Yilei Mao and colleagues administered two species of probiotic bacteria (lactobacilli) to mice with severe colitis, induced by a drug, methotrexate. Half the mice also received oat fibre that had been fermented by the lactobacilli. All the mice had reduced severity of disease, but those receiving the oat fibre, in addition to the probiotic bacteria, fared better.[19]

Karen Madsen and colleagues administered *Lactobacillus reuteri* bacteria rectally to mice with colitis that had decreased levels of lactobacillus bacteria. Normalising these levels reduced other types of bacteria and prevented colitis.[20] In a later study, Madsen used the same type of mice (IL10-gene deficient) with a 'cocktail' of probiotic bacteria (VSL#3), and a significant reduction in colitis was achieved.[21]

At least five other studies of probiotics on colitis in mice and rats have been published as abstracts (summaries). All of these also showed significant reduction in disease.

While a great deal can be learned from animal studies, mouse models of colitis are not identical to UC and Crohn's.[22] Ultimately a proposed treatment for humans has to be tried out on humans.

Clinical trials

In an early study[23] a patient with troublesome UC was given a short course of antibiotics to kill off colonic bacteria and then given an enema of faecal material from a healthy donor. This produced remission of symptoms, but as Cummings and Macfarlane commented, "this treatment is understandably difficult to sell to patients".[3]

The 1990s brought more studies, with larger groups of patients. Wolfgang Kruis and colleagues compared the use of mesalazine (a drug commonly used for colitis) to a beneficial strain of *Escherichia coli*, *E. coli* Nissle 1917, in 120 people with inactive UC. The 12-week randomised controlled trial revealed no significant differences in disease activity, relapse rates and relapse-free time. The authors concluded that probiotic treatment might offer another option for maintenance therapy in UC.[24]

B. J. Rembacken and colleagues administered *E. coli* Nissle 1917 to 57 people with active UC, and compared results with 59 people treated with mesalazine. Both groups received standard medical therapy as well, until remission was achieved, and patients were maintained on either treatment (mesalazine or probiotic) for a maximum of 12 months. In the mesalazine group, 44 (75%) attained remission, and of these, 32 (73%) relapsed after one year. In the probiotic group, 39 (68%) remitted, and of these, 26 (67%) relapsed after one year. The authors concluded that the *E. coli* strain may have an effect equal to that of mesalazine in maintaining remission in UC. It is not clear what effect the probiotic had in helping to achieve remission, because standard medical therapy was used at the same time.[25]

The evidence from the two studies above by Kruis and by Rembacken was reinforced by a later study. This involved 222 patients with UC in remission, comparing *E. coli* Nissle 1917 and mesalazine. After one year, the study found that relapses occurred in 36% of those receiving the probiotic and 33% of those receiving the mesalazine.[26]

E. coli Nissle 1917 has also been used with colonic Crohn's patients in a small study by Helmut Malchow. The randomised controlled trial involved 28 patients and lasted a year. All of the participants received steroids to promote remission, and one group also received the probiotic. During the year, the reduction in the use of steroids by the probiotic group was substantially greater than in the control group; and after one year, a third of the probiotic group had relapsed compared with two-thirds of the control group.[27]

Alessandro Venturi and colleagues reported on a new probiotic preparation in 1999, VSL#3 (VSL Pharmaceuticals Inc.), which contains three strains of bifidobacteria, four strains of lactobacilli, and *Streptococcus thermophilus*. In a small study, 20 patients who could not tolerate the UC treatment 5-ASA were treated with VSL#3 for 12 months. The probiotic strains of bacteria increased in the intestine, as measured in faecal samples. Fifteen of the 20 remained in remission. The authors suggested that this treatment might be useful in maintaining remission in people with UC who cannot take 5-ASA, but controlled trials would be necessary to confirm these effects.[28]

Paolo Gionchetti and colleagues evaluated VSL#3 in 40 people with pouchitis, administering the treatment or an inactive placebo for nine months. Three patients (15%) in the VSL#3 group relapsed, compared with 20 (100%) in the placebo group. This study suggests a use for VSL#3 in preventing pouchitis relapse.[29]

Mario Guslandi and his colleagues conducted research on 32 Crohn's patients in remission. Half received the normal dose of mesalazine (also known as mesalamine). The other group received mesalazine plus the yeast *Saccharomyces boulardii*. After six months, only one of the sixteen receiving the yeast had relapsed, while six out of sixteen of the mesalazine-only group had relapsed.[30]

How strong is the above evidence?

While the above trials in patients with IBD seem to have confirmed the promising effects of probiotics seen in animal models,[1] a majority of the reviewers felt that the clinical evidence was not yet strong enough to be completely convincing.

Fergus Shanahan commented that "Enthusiasm for probiotics in IBD is strong on rationale and preclinical data but still weak on rigorous evidence for clinical efficacy".[7] Faubion and Sandborn felt it was still too soon to recommend routine use of probiotics in general clinical practice.[2] And Jeffrey Katz and Claudio Fiocchi concluded that "These exciting initial studies strongly support the use of probiotic formulas in the treatment of IBD", but added that "preliminary results do not yet prove that probiotics can successfully treat IBD other than pouchitis".[8] They felt that more rigorous research, in the form of larger controlled trials, was necessary.

Although current evidence does not support the use of probiotics as a routine part of medical treatment, the growing body of research and the wide availability of products warrant a thorough review of what is known about specific probiotic microbes.

Chapter summary

- In surgery for Crohn's Disease of the colon, if the faecal stream is diverted then the inflammation usually diminishes. The inflammation is likely to return, however, when the flow of faeces is reconnected.

- An ileo-anal pouch (formed in UC patients after surgical removal of the colon), develops large numbers of bacteria and it is quite common for pouchitis (inflammation of the pouch) to appear. This is surprising because the pouch is made from small intestine and patients with UC do not have inflammation in the small intestine.

- Mice which would normally have colitis (because of feed or gene alteration) do not have the inflammation if they are germ-free (kept in a sterile environment or treated with antibiotics).

- There is growing evidence that people with IBD have intestinal flora that are different from healthy people.

- Feeding probiotic bacteria to mice with colitis has led to the prevention or control of colitis.

- There have been a small number of trials of probiotics on people with UC, pouchitis and Crohn's, with encouraging results. The evidence is not yet sufficient, however, for probiotics to become routine medical treatment for IBD.

5. Specific Species & Strains

"I have had proctitis for more than forty years, and four years ago I started taking an acidophilus capsule once a day. The effects have been less inflammation in the rectum, less pain, less wind and mucus, less urgency to find a toilet when out and about, which is a blessing in itself, more energy, and less need to use medication for proctitis. My doctor approves of the fact that I am taking probiotics."

This chapter lists specific probiotic species and strains that have been tested on people with IBD and other intestinal diseases, and describes the evidence of benefit for each type of probiotic.

The naming system

To understand the differences between various probiotic bacteria it helps to know how bacteria are classified, that is, how they are grouped and named.

Just as many of us have a family name and two personal names, so scientists have given bacteria three names.

Rather like the Chinese naming system where the family name comes first, the bacterial family name, known as the **genus**, comes first. The two genus names that constitute the majority of probiotics (as currently understood) are *Lactobacillus* and *Bifidobacterium*. Genera (the plural of genus) are agreed by scientists on the basis of shared characteristics, for example, shape, behaviour, genes.

The second part of the name is called the **species**. A well-known probiotic species is acidophilus. A species name is never properly used except with the genus name. Thus *Lactobacillus acidophilus* is a proper species name (sometimes abbreviated to *L. acidophilus*).

The third part of the name is the **strain** (or variety). Bacterial strains can vary in very small ways from other strains in the same species. These tiny differences can sometimes mean major differences in their characteristics. The strain name comes after the genus and species names and may be letters, numbers, a combination of these or occasionally a word or name.

A good way of remembering the importance of strains is to think of *Escherichia coli* (often abbreviated to *E. coli*). Many people will have heard of *E. coli* as a source of serious food poisoning, which can lead to death in vulnerable people. But, as we learned in the previous chapter, one of the better-documented bacterial treatments of IBD is *E. coli*.

The difference is the strain. The majority of cases of food poisoning are caused by *E. coli* O157. The probiotic strain is called *E. coli* Nissle 1917.

Strain differences are found in various parts of bacteria.

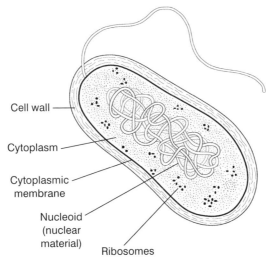

Cell wall

Cytoplasm

Cytoplasmic membrane

Nucleoid (nuclear material)

Ribosomes

Fig 7. The main parts of a bacterium

Escherichia coli Nissle 1917

This probiotic has shown benefits in several studies involving more than 450 patients with UC and a small number with Crohn's.[1] These studies took place at the turn of the twenty-first century, but there is a longer history to this probiotic.

History

The *E. coli* species was identified in 1885 by the German paediatrician Professor Theodor Escherich. He named it *Bacterium coli commune*, but in 1919 (eight years after his death) the species was renamed *Escherichia coli*.

Another German physician, Professor Alfred Nissle, identified the Nissle 1917 strain. He became interested in the 'antagonism' of some strains of *E. coli* against pathogenic intestinal bacteria.

During the First World War he visited field hospitals and took stool samples from soldiers who were unaffected by intestinal infections, a major cause of illness among the troops. In laboratory tests he compared the different strains for their ability to suppress the growth of typhoid bacteria.[2]

The type that he found most effective in its antagonistic actions was named the Nissle strain, which he isolated from the stool of a non-commissioned officer in Dobruja, south-eastern Europe. Nissle grew this strain of bacteria and added it to gelatine capsules, sealed with wax or paraffin. He tested the bacterial capsule on himself with no negative effects, and started manufacturing it under the name Mutaflor (flora-changing) in 1917.

Production of Mutaflor has continued almost uninterrupted since then. The current product has an added enteric coating, so that the Nissle bacteria are protected against stomach acid and are not released until the capsule reaches the ileum and colon.

Why does E. coli Nissle 1917 help UC and Crohn's?

It is not obvious why a probiotic bacterium that protects against infectious diarrhoea should also help with UC and Crohn's. Infectious diarrhoea and IBD are different conditions; additionally IBD is not infectious. Even though *E. coli* Nissle 1917 has been found to be helpful in IBD, it is not known for certain how it works.

One of the teams that undertook a large study of UC and *E. coli* Nissle 1917 theorised that the probiotic may work by occupying space on the intestinal wall which might otherwise be occupied by harmful bacteria.[3]

Some bacterial species produce antimicrobial substances (bacteriocins) that help them to remain viable in the intestine by killing or inhibiting other bacteria. *E. coli* strains produce various bacteriocins (called colicins) that are active against other *E. coli* strains.[4] Perhaps, therefore, *E. coli* Nissle 1917 may work by producing chemicals that attack pathogenic *E. coli* and thus make it easier for the probiotic to replace the pathogen on the gut wall.

Various studies have shown that harmful forms of *E. coli* are associated with IBD. For example, Mary Cooke showed, in her examination of stool samples, that patients with UC had a higher proportion of pathogenic strains of *E. coli* than people with infectious diarrhoea, or those with no intestinal disease. She also found that a larger proportion of *E. coli* from UC patients was resistant to antibiotic treatment.[5]

M. Giaffer and colleagues described several studies that showed more of the strains of *E. coli* found in people with IBD were those that attached to the gut wall (enteroadherent). In addition, Giaffer's own study found that 62% of patients with Crohn's and 68% of those with UC had enteroadherent *E. coli*, compared with only 6% of healthy people.[6]

Genus *Lactobacillus*

The majority of the species available in probiotic products are from the genus *Lactobacillus*.

Part of the reason for this popularity is historical. The bacterium favoured by Metchnikoff (see Chapter 2) in the early twentieth century was a lactobacillus. That species is the same or similar to that used in yoghurt production, which has a long history of safe consumption.

Also, lactobacilli are relatively easy to produce on an industrial scale, as shown by the dairy industry.[2]

Another reason is the evidence of lactobacilli exerting a controlling effect on harmful *E. coli* reducing their numbers.[7]

Subsequent research and farming experience has supported the initial belief in the suitability of some lactobacillus species as probiotics.

Beneficial species and strains

Reviews identify three strains of lactobacilli that have been shown to have positive effects on people with IBD: *L. salivarius* UCC118, *L. plantarum* 299v and *L. rhamnosus* GG (the last sometimes also known as *L. casei* GG or *L.* GG).[1,8] However, all of the four studies involved, however, were weak methodologically (for example, small numbers, no control group).

When good results from studies on mouse models of colitis are also considered, plus evidence of probiotics working on other intestinal diseases, a list can be produced of lactobacilli strains for which there is some scientific evidence of health benefit:

L. rhamnosus GG (ATCC 53103)

L. plantarum 299 and 299v

L. salivarius UCC118

L. reuteri

L. acidophilus NFCO (or NCDO) 1748

L. johnsonii La1 (also known as LC-1 or LJ-1)

L. casei Shirota

L. casei DN-114 001

The list covers seven different species of lactobacilli (rhamnosus, plantarum, salivarius, reuteri, acidophilus, johnsonii, and casei). While strains of the same species may have some characteristics that are distinctly different from each other, it is also true that bacteria of the same species usually share a large number of the same characteristics.

How do lactobacilli work probiotically?

As with *E. coli* Nissle 1917, it is not known for certain how lactobacilli might work as probiotic bacteria. There are several possible explanations, all of which may contribute to the probiotic effect, depending on the type of species and strain, and depending on the local ecology (interrelationship) of the gut and bacteria.

The most likely explanations for the probiotic effect of lactobacilli are that they:

- increase the acidity
- strengthen the intestinal cell barrier
- produce antibiotic-like substances and other chemicals
- fill adhesion sites and thus exclude pathogens
- promote larger quantities of intestinal mucus

These factors are explained more fully below.

The main product of the fermentation of carbohydrates by lactobacilli is lactic acid. 'Lactic acid bacteria' is a term used to describe a number of bacterial genera, including the lactobacilli. It has been argued that the lactic acid lowers the pH (that is, it increases acidity) of the ileum and colon and that this discourages harmful bacteria. In addition, other acids, known as short-chain fatty acids (SCFAs), are produced by the fermentation process and may also make the area more acidic.

Some of the SCFAs are known to be consumed by the enterocytes (gut wall cells), which are likely to be strengthened as a consequence. Healthy enterocytes can reduce the translocation (passage) of microbes through the lining of the intestine into the bloodstream. When a 'leaky gut' is repaired, overstimulation of the immune system by microbes may be reduced.

There have been reports of lactobacilli producing antibiotic-like substances called bacteriocins, which may help to restrict the growth of intestinal pathogens.[9] Also, some lactic acid bacteria produce hydrogen peroxide, a chemical that has an antibacterial effect. More is produced in the small intestine than in the colon, as the bacteria need oxygen for the chemical process involved.

Some microbiologists believe that adhesion to the gut wall, even for a short time, is the key factor in excluding potentially harmful bacteria. Effective probiotic lactobacilli tend to be good at attaching to the mucosa (mucus-covered intestinal lining).[10]

Some probiotic lactobacilli stimulate the extra production of mucus by gut wall cells, and this may be a way in which the lactobacilli inhibit the attachment of pathogenic bacteria.[11]

L. bulgaricus

L. bulgaricus, the bacterium associated with Metchnikoff (see Chapter 2), does not appear in the list of lactobacilli that have shown significant probiotic benefits. The reason for this is that many researchers have shown that L. bulgaricus is very poor at surviving the effect of stomach acid. The L. bulgaricus bacteria that do survive do not attach to the wall of the lower intestine and therefore are less likely to influence the intestine. The same is true of Streptococcus thermophilus, another bacterium used as a starter culture for yoghurt.

This does not mean that there are no benefits from consuming yoghurt. The yoghurt bacteria may have effects as they pass through the intestine and beneficial chemicals may be produced in the yoghurt as a result of the fermentation. In the context of bacterial strains that have been shown to have direct benefits on health, however, neither *L. bulgaricus* nor *S. thermophilus* are in this category, based on current knowledge.

Genus *Bifidobacterium*

Bifidobacteria are the second largest group of probiotic species, and are commonly added to fermented milk products in Europe.

Like lactobacilli, bifidobacteria produce lactic acid, although they are from a branch of bacteria distinct from the lactobacilli and other 'lactic acid bacteria'.

Their difference is demonstrated in two ways.

First, the shape: bacteria are found in two main forms; bead-shaped (cocci) and rod-shaped (bacilli). Bifidobacteria are different, however, as they are usually Y-shaped. Their name comes from 'bifidus', meaning split in two parts.

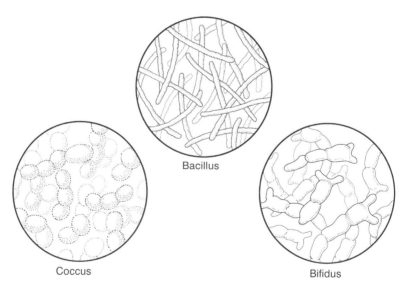

Bacillus

Coccus

Bifidus

Fig 8. Coccus, bacillus and bifidus shapes of bacteria

Another difference of the bifidobacterium family is that they produce acetic acid, that is in vinegar, in addition to lactic acid.

Why have bifidobacteria been chosen as probiotics?

There are two main reasons why bifidobacteria have been selected for probiotic products.

First, their presence in very large numbers in babies of a few days old has provided reassurance that they are not harmful. It was in 1899 that Henry Tissier of the Pasteur Institute, when examining the faeces of a baby, became the first to identify the unusual shaped microbe which later became known as *Bifidobacterium*. Research in the second half of the twentieth century has shown that bifidobacteria become the dominant bacterium in infant intestines when the baby is about one week old, increasing to as much as 90 per cent of the microflora. From weaning onwards their numbers and proportions fall towards the normal adult mixture.[12]

Secondly, unlike the two starter cultures used in yoghurts, bifidobacteria are resistant to acid and have good survival rates in their passage through the stomach.

How might bifidobacteria work?

Acetic acid, together with lactic acid, may lower the pH (increasing acidity) in local areas of the gut.

In the adult human gut, bifidobacteria are, on average, seven times more common than lactobacilli and are present in very large numbers. They constitute about 5 per cent of all known gut bacteria.[13] It is possible, therefore, that their ability to increase the acidity of the intestine, together with their large numbers in the intestine, may be a factor in their probiotic effects, as many harmful microbes are inhibited in a low pH environment.

There is also some limited evidence that bifidobacteria produce anti-bacterial substances that inhibit harmful bacteria. Eight such species showed this effect in laboratory experiments, the most effective being *Bif. infantis* NCFB2205 and *Bif. longum* NCFB2259.[4] The anti-bacterial substances have not yet been identified but may be similar to the bacteriocins produced by lactobacilli.

Other useful characteristics of bifidobacteria are the production of various B vitamins, and a tendency to adhere well to the intestinal wall, thus excluding pathogenic bacteria.[14]

Evidence of probiotic effects

Bearing in mind that it is increasingly common for bifidobacteria to be added to fermented milk products (for example, bio-yoghurts), it is surprising how limited the research evidence is for the beneficial health effects of this group of bacteria.

There is some research evidence which points to bifidobacteria digesting lactose (milk sugar), reducing cholesterol levels, reducing diarrhoea and improving the immune system. The evidence is nevertheless very limited.

There have been some probiotic studies in which bifidobacteria have been part of a mixture of several species of bacteria, usually lactobacilli. Therefore, it has not been possible to identify which species have actually worked. These studies included two small studies on IBD patients, but there have been no probiotic studies on IBD patients involving only bifidobacteria.

Classification

Another problem with evidence for the benefit of bifidobacteria is taxonomy (classification).

There has been a difficulty in classifying bacteria. Historically, bacteria have been grouped and named according to their shape and other physical characteristics, their behaviour and their preferred habitats. As knowledge of bacteria has increased, however, species have been renamed. This process has accelerated since bacteria have been analysed using genetic and molecular methods. For instance, as stated previously, *L. rhamnosus* GG used to be known as *L. casei* GG.

The classification problem is particularly severe with the genus of bifidobacterium. For example, *Bif. lactis* used to be known as *Bif. bifidum*, and before that *Bif. animalis*. And on some occasions *Bif. longum*.[15] It can therefore sometimes be unclear which species has been tested, particularly in earlier studies where classification was less precise.

Currently, thirty species of bifidobacteria have been firmly identified and now there is considerable potential for investigating the species and strains that have the strongest probiotic effects. At present, however, for people with IBD there is very little reliable information as to which particular bifidobacteria might be helpful to them.

Other probiotics

Several other types of microbes are used in probiotic products for humans.

Bacillus subtilis

Bacillus subtilis is a soil organism, which is mostly used in animal preparations. It can form spores (a hard coating to protect against dehydration) and the probiotic products tend to use the spore form. As such, it is more likely to survive its passage through stomach acid.

Roy Fuller (who produced the first widely-accepted definition of probiotics) has, however, questioned the value of *Bacillus subtilis*. He commented that "it is difficult to see how this can be active in the gut; it is certainly not an intestinal organism and, since it is a strict aerobe [needs oxygen], would not be able to grow or metabolise in the gut".[7]

Some scientists argue that it is better to use human-derived microbes, because they are more likely to be safe and are more likely to adhere to the human gut wall.

Saccharomyces boulardii

One of the non-human probiotics that has been regularly used in humans is a yeast (a type of fungus), *Saccharomyces boulardii*.

In addition to the positive results in the study with Crohn's patients by Guslandi, as reported in Chapter 4, *S. boulardii* has also been shown to be effective in reducing and preventing diarrhoea from a variety of causes. Piero Periti and F. Tonelli reviewed twelve randomised controlled trials carried out between 1976 and 1995. They reported that "The efficacy of this yeast has been demonstrated on a total of 2,581 patients for various indications including the prevention of traveller's diarrhoea (n=1,231), antibiotic or enteral feeding-associated diarrhoea (n=929), treatment of acute or chronic diarrhoea in adults, children or AIDS patients (n=297), and the recurrence of *C. difficile* colitis (n=124)".[16] [In this quotation, n= the number of patients studied].

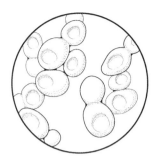

Fig 9. Saccharomyces boulardii

The French scientist H. Boulard first identified the yeast *S. boulardii* in the 1920s. He had observed that people in Indochina traditionally treated diarrhoea with an extract from the shells of lychee fruit. The yeast from these shells was manufactured in Europe from the 1950s, and in freeze-dried form from the 1960s. It is available in some European, South American and African countries and in the USA.

Worms

A microbe that has been tested on one group of people with IBD is helminth worms.

Trichuris suis is a parasitic whipworm found in pigs, and is known to reduce the level of response in the mucosal immune system by affecting the T-helper cells. Researchers in the University of Iowa wanted to find out if they might be beneficial in treating IBD. Six patients with hard-to-treat IBD (four with Crohn's, two with UC) took a single dose of 2,500 microscopic parasite eggs. The eggs hatched into worms in the intestines and all six patients experienced significant improvements; for example, there were many fewer bowel movements.

Although the worms were similar to a human whipworm, they were sufficiently different not to become established in the gut, and all were excreted after approximately one month.[17]

Shanahan commented that "the lack of immunologic exposure to helminths in Westernized societies might, in part, account for some of the rise in the prevalence of CD [Crohn's Disease]".[18] Hygenic surroundings have reduced mortality and improved health generally, but at the same time the development of a fully functioning immune system may be impaired. Worms and other parasites may dampen some aspects of the mucosal immune response. It is suggested that without these parasitic worms the human body may over-produce powerful substances that cause excessive inflammation.

It should be remembered, however, that the worms experiment was a pilot study involving very few participants and no controls. Worms are not currently available in any commercial product.

Genus Enterococcus

Enterococcus is one of a group of genera, including *Lactobacillus*, known as 'lactic acid bacteria'. The most common species used as a probiotic is *Ent. faecium* (formerly known as *Streptococcus faecium*), and within that species the most commonly used strain is SF68. There have been no studies on IBD with this probiotic; almost all of the reported studies have been on infectious diarrhoea. For example, in a randomised study of 21 adults with acute diarrhoea, by the third day only 8% of those taking the SF68 strain still had diarrhoea, compared with 66% in the placebo group.[19]

Unlike other lactic acid bacteria, however, there are growing safety concerns about enterococci, particularly *Ent. faecium* and *Ent. faecalis*, as a possible cause of antibiotic-resistant infections in hospitals. On the other hand, there is no evidence of anyone developing an infection from taking a probiotic product containing enterococci.[20]

Safety

As some microbes cause disease, it is reasonable to ask whether probiotics are safe.

In a review of safety, experts from nine European countries reported that "lactic-acid bacteria in foods have a long history of safe use".[21]

While lactobacillus and bifidobacterium species are generally recognised as being very safe, no bacterium is completely safe, whatever its species. In certain circumstances, particularly when tissues are damaged or when the host has a severely weakened immune system, any bacterium may act in an invasive and potentially harmful way. This should be born in mind by people with IBD, who may be prescribed immune suppressing drugs and may have sores on the gut wall and wounds from intestinal surgery. Having said this, illness arising from probiotic products is virtually unknown.

For a more detailed description about the safety of probiotics, see Appendix 2.

Is there hope for a clearer picture?

Having reviewed current knowledge on probiotic species and strains for IBD, it may seem somewhat limited. Will people with UC and Crohn's have to wait for another decade until research has uncovered more information about probiotic bacteria? Thankfully, there have been two notable recent developments.

First, the European Union has funded a major multi-centred programme of research into probiotics, entitled PROEUHEALTH. Part of this programme is to examine the effects of two probiotic strains on IBD. Co-ordinated by Professor Fergus Shanahan of Cork University, Ireland, it involves researchers from four other European countries (for details see: www.vtt.fi).

At the same time, an independent company (VSL Pharmaceuticals Inc., Ft. Lauderdale, FL) has developed a product, VSL#3, consisting of eight bacterial species, that is being tested in several centres in North America, Europe and Asia.

VSL#3 contains three species of lactobacilli, four species of bifidobacteria and a streptococcus, as a freeze-dried powder of 450 billion bacteria per sachet. The strains are of long-standing use in the dairy industry and therefore have an especially good safety profile.

Two of the studies on people with IBD, reported in Chapter 4, used VSL#3, and encouraging results were achieved.

Other IBD-related studies using VSL#3, yet to report, include maintenance of remission in Crohn's, treatment of mild active UC, as well as a study to reduce the use of steroids in children. Further information on these studies can be found on the company's web site (www.vslpharma.com).

Chapter summary

- Bacteria have three parts to their name: genus, species and strain. The full name is important in correctly identifying the content of a probiotic product.

- *E. coli* Nissle 1917 has been commercially available since the 1920s. It may work in replacing or keeping at bay harmful strains of *E. coli* that have been shown to be present in greater numbers in people with IBD.

- Lactobacillus species are the most common group of probiotic bacteria. Several species have shown benefits for people with IBD, but in very limited studies.

- A list of lactobacillus strains was produced for which there is some scientific evidence of health benefit with IBD or other intestinal conditions.

- Lactobacillus probiotics may work through increasing acidity, reducing gut permeability, producing anti-bacterial substances, filling adhesion sites and stimulating mucus production.

- Bifidobacteria are an important part of the normal gut flora and some species from this genus form the second most commonly used group of probiotic bacteria.

- There is no research evidence that clearly supports benefit for IBD by bifidobacteria, but there is evidence of other health benefits.

- Other microbes used in probiotic products include three that do not normally reside in human intestines. They are *Bacillus subtilis* (soil-based and used mostly in farmed animals), *Saccharomyces boulardii* (a yeast for which there is limited evidence of benefit for IBD) and *Trichuris suis* (a parasitic worm for which there is preliminary evidence of benefit for people with IBD).

- Enterococci are occasionally used as probiotics. Unlike other lactic-acid bacteria, there are some concerns over the safety of enterococci. There is no evidence, however, of anyone developing an infection from enterococci in a probiotic product.

- Lactobacilli and bifidobacteria are very safe, but no bacteria are completely safe, particularly if you are in a physically weak state. Further information on safety can be found in Appendix 2.

- The European Union has funded a major programme of research on probiotics (PROEUHEALTH) and this may provide new information on a range of issues, including treatment of IBD.

- VSL#3 is a probiotic product, consisting of a cocktail of eight species of bacteria in very large numbers. IBD-related research into this product has been very encouraging and further research on IBD patients using VSL#3 is continuing.

6. *Prebiotics* – What Are They?

"I have been taking home-made yoghurt, with added probiotic bacteria and prebiotics, for one year, and in the last six months have taken no medication at all after gradually decreasing it under hospital supervision. At my last inspection the colitis had all but disappeared. I am not saying it will work for everybody, but it has thankfully worked for me. I am a completely new person."

So far, this book has described how the effects of the bacteria in the gut may be improved by adding probiotic bacteria. The gut, however, also contains food, both whole and broken down. Can the gut bacteria be improved by changing the food we eat? This is the thinking behind *pre*biotics.

What are *pre*biotics?

*Pre*biotics are food ingredients and supplements that encourage the growth of beneficial bacteria whilst having a neutral or negative effect on harmful bacteria.

In the second half of the twentieth century in Europe some products were described as 'bifidogenic', that is, they stimulated the growth of bifidobacteria. It was not until 1995, however, that Glenn Gibson and Marcel Roberfroid introduced the term '*prebiotics*'. Their definition is, "non-digestible food ingredients that beneficially affect the host by selectively stimulating the growth and/or activity of one or a limited number of bacteria in the colon, that can improve host health".[1]

*Pre*biotics are important to the idea of improving IBD with probiotics, because they complement probiotic bacteria and may strengthen their effectiveness.

As most food is broken down and absorbed into the body in the small intestine, is there any left for bacteria to use in the lower intestine?

We pass bodily waste as stools (faeces), so there does seem to be something that is undigested. Of the solid matter in the stools, approximately 55 per cent is bacterial cells (either live or dead).[2] There is also a small amount of waste from the intestine itself, for example, sloughed gut wall cells, mucus, digestive enzymes. The remaining part of faeces is food that has not been digested.

Bacteria 'feed' on undigested food through the process of fermentation, which involves breaking down the food particles into smaller compounds and releasing energy and gases.

Food consists of three main elements: protein, for building body tissues; carbohydrates, for energy; and fats, for storing energy. Which of the three types of food might be prebiotic? In theory, all might be, as they can all be fermented. In practice, however, all known prebiotic products have been certain types of carbohydrates, because probiotic types of bacteria easily ferment them.

The main types of prebiotic carbohydrate are known as non-digestible oligosaccharides (NDOs).

Non-digestible oligosaccharides (NDOs)

NDOs are a form of dietary fibre. Many people are familiar with the idea that dietary fibre is good for digestive health because it reduces constipation and haemorrhoids, as well as the risk of colon cancer and heart disease.

Dietary fibre can be divided into two categories: insoluble and soluble. Insoluble fibre mostly comprises plant cell walls. In addition to not being digested in the small intestine, most insoluble fibre is not fermented in the colon, either.

In comparison, NDOs are a type of soluble fibre that is found in the main body of some plants, where they act as a carbohydrate store. The fact that NDOs can dissolve in water means that bacteria find them much easier to ferment.

NDOs are non-digestible. The enzymes and other chemicals produced by the body to break down food do not work on this type of carbohydrate. Thus NDOs reach the lower part of the gut where most of the bacteria are to be found.

6: Prebiotics – What Are They?

'Oligo' means few and a saccharide is a sugar, so an oligosaccharide is a carbohydrate that is made up of a small number of sugar molecules linked together. The way in which sugars are linked together determines whether or not they are digestible.

How do NDOs work?

The way NDOs work appears to be two-fold. First, they encourage the growth of beneficial bacteria, and secondly, they attract harmful bacteria away from the mucosa (mucus-lined gut wall).

Boosting beneficial bacteria

The majority of bacterial species in the colon are saccharolytic (ferment carbohydrates), including the probiotic bifidobacteria and lactobacilli.[3] In comparison, many harmful bacteria are proteolytic (ferment protein) and some of these do not ferment any carbohydrates.

This might suggest that all that is needed to achieve a healthier bacterial balance is to increase the amount of carbohydrate in the colon, which in turn would boost the numbers of the saccharolytic bacteria. However, some saccharolytic bacteria are more beneficial than others, and it is necessary to target the best by selecting particular carbohydrates for the *pre*biotic purpose.

While there are other carbohydrates that are not digested in the small intestine, for example, resistant starch, it is the NDOs that seem to be the most effective in stimulating the growth of probiotic bacteria. In particular, NDOs help to increase the numbers of bifidobacteria, which tend to be very efficient at fermenting NDOs.

One study showed that bifidobacteria and lactobacilli respond faster than other bacteria to the NDO lactulose.[4] In another study, the consumption of 12.5g per day for 12 days of the NDO oligofructose (FOS) increased the number of bifidobacteria ten-fold.[5]

One benefit of boosting bifidobacterial numbers is increased acidity, arising from the production of acetic and lactic acid, which can inhibit undesirable bacteria.

It is not fully known why bifidobacteria respond to NDOs, but it may be that bifidobacteria produce enzymes that are especially effective in breaking NDOs into smaller molecules and releasing energy that bifidobacteria then use to grow and reproduce.

In the mid-1990s, the European Commission funded a multinational research project (ENDO) into NDOs, and in 1998, the researchers summarised the current state of knowledge.[6]

One of their conclusions was that the bifidogenic effect of a *pre*biotic NDO is inversely related to a person's initial count of bifidobacteria. This means that *pre*biotics do not seem to increase the numbers of bifidobacteria very much if those numbers are already at a high level. But they are very effective if the person taking the *pre*biotic NDO starts with low numbers of bifidobacteria.

As the numbers of bifidobacteria and lactobacilli are low in Crohn's patients (and severe cases of UC), the bacterial balance could be brought closer to that of healthy people by the use of *pre*biotic NDOs that boost the numbers of bifidobacteria and lactobacilli.

Anti-adhesive properties

Pathogenic bacteria use proteins (for example, adhesin) to attach themselves to carbohydrates, which are an integral part of the surface of human cells. This locking mechanism helps bacteria to become more secure and start disease processes, for example, through producing toxins.

Carbohydrate taken as food can also attach to harmful bacteria and, as a consequence, can decoy these bacteria away from epithelial cells lining the gut wall, by offering a large number of alternative carbohydrate attachments.

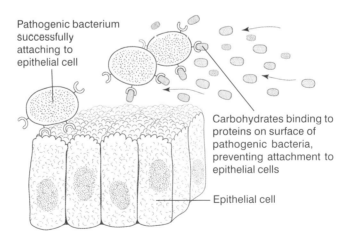

Pathogenic bacterium successfully attaching to epithelial cell

Carbohydrates binding to proteins on surface of pathogenic bacteria, preventing attachment to epithelial cells

Epithelial cell

Fig 10. Mechanisms whereby certain types of carbohydrate may prevent pathogens from attaching to epithelial cells.

6: Prebiotics – What Are They?

The carbohydrates that seem to be most effective in this process are soluble oligosaccharides, including NDOs.[7,8] The benefits of breast-milk in reducing the risk of infection to babies in the first year of their life is believed to be due, in part, to the oligosaccharides in the milk stopping harmful bacteria from becoming established.

For people with Crohn's or UC, the relevance of this effect is that NDOs might have the added benefit of removing some of the many bacteria that attach to the mucosa in IBD, which may be a factor in the cause or continuation of IBD.

Evidence of *pre*biotic benefit in IBD

Several studies provide evidence of *pre*biotic benefit for IBD. One study found that the use of a *pre*biotic, lactulose, was as effective as *Lactobacillus reuteri* in reducing symptoms of colitis in mice.[9] In another, a *pre*biotic, inulin, reduced inflammation in rats with colitis.[10]

In a human trial, using the *pre*biotic lactosucrose, seven patients, two with Crohn's and the rest with UC, consumed 8.5g of lactosucrose syrup each day for a fortnight. An examination of faecal samples showed that bifidobacteria were found in all seven patients after 14 days of lactosucrose consumption, while only three patients had bifidobacteria at a measurable level at the beginning of the research. Among those three who already had the bifidobacteria, however, there was no significant change in the bifidobacterial numbers.

This study supports the idea that *pre*biotics are most helpful when bifidobacteria are relatively low in number. It also shows that the number of lactobacilli increased ten-fold, on average, after a fortnight of receiving the lactosucrose.

Furthermore, bowel movements improved in four out of the seven patients.[11] As all the patients were on low-residue, low-fat diets, except for one who was on an elemental diet (liquid nutrition), it seems that the *pre*biotic helped to get the right balance between constipation and diarrhoea.

A randomised controlled trial was undertaken on 19 patients with ileo-anal pouches. They received 24g of the *pre*biotic inulin daily for three weeks, and a placebo at another time (a crossover study). It was a double-blind study, in that neither the patient nor the researcher knew which was the inulin and which was the placebo. The inulin supplementation led to a reduction in inflammation of the mucosa (lining) of the pouches compared with the placebo.[12]

These studies do provide some encouragement for the idea that *prebiotics* can be of practical benefit to people with IBD, but much more research is needed to prove safety and effectiveness. For example, it is not clear what other genera of bacteria, in addition to bifidobacteria and lactobacilli, may be stimulated by *prebiotics* and what effect this may have on health.

Gas production

The main side effect reported by people participating in NDO *prebiotic* trials is an increase in gas production, resulting in more flatulence and sometimes uncomfortable bloating.

For example, there were noticeable increases in flatulence among 64 healthy young women, who were taking part in a study consuming 14g daily of the *prebiotic* inulin (as part of a low-fat spread). The increase in gas production was usually described as mild, but 12 per cent of the participants described the discomfort as 'severe'.[13]

As bifidobacteria and lactobacilli produce no gas in their fermentation of carbohydrates, why should increased gas production be a problem with NDOs? It is almost certainly because other bacteria in the microflora are fermenting some of the NDOs and consequently producing gas.

In theory, it should be possible to control the excess gas. As bifidobacteria are the most efficient type of intestinal bacteria in fermenting NDOs, the more bifidobacteria there are, the less *prebiotic* will be left for gas-producing bacteria to ferment. Therefore, if less NDO is taken when there are fewer bifidobacteria present and then steadily increased as the bifidobacteria increase in numbers, there should be very little spare NDO for other bacteria to use.

This theory is supported by the clinical experience of some dieticians and nutritionists who have found that gas production can be managed by gradually increasing the amount of fibre in the diet.

Furthermore, one study of six healthy volunteers taking 20g per day of the NDO oligofructose for 11 days found no gas problems. The NDO had been introduced gradually, starting with a quarter of the dose and steadily increasing it.[14]

Another way of controlling gas may be in the choice of *prebiotic*. There is some indication that different *prebiotics* lead to different levels of gas production. For example, the *prebiotic* inulin may produce above-average amounts of gas compared with other NDOs, while another *prebiotic*, TOS, may produce less than average. Current evidence as to which NDOs create the least gas, however, is too limited to be a reliable guide. (See Chapter 7 for a more extensive discussion of different types of *prebiotics*.)

Advantages of *prebiotics*

The main advantage of *prebiotics* is that they can increase the numbers of beneficial bacteria already present in the microflora, rather than trying to introduce new bacterial strains, as with probiotics.

Prebiotics can also be used in probiotic products to strengthen the probiotic bacteria by providing them with readily available food that they are able to ferment.

Unlike some probiotics, which have to be stored carefully (for example, refrigerated) and have a shelf life of only a few months, *prebiotics* do not have any significant storage problems. This is because they do not have live contents.

Another advantage is that some *prebiotics* occur naturally in plants and therefore may be seen to be part of a normal diet. Increasingly, food companies are using NDOs in their products. They are used to replace sugar and fat, to add bulk, and to improve the texture of the food without adding substantially to its calorific value.

Food companies are also attracted to the idea that NDOs have the potential to turn their products into 'functional foods', where health benefits are found in addition to the usual nutritional benefits. Manufactured food products are therefore likely to appear that identify *prebiotic* NDOs in their contents.

The cost of producing NDOs is relatively low compared with probiotics, because of large-scale demand from food companies and because NDOs are much easier to manufacture than probiotics.

The potential for greater profits for food companies through the promotion of 'functional foods' (also known as nutraceuticals) means that funds are likely to be made available for more research into NDO *prebiotics*.

Chapter summary

- *Prebiotics* are "non-digestible food ingredients that beneficially affect the host by selectively stimulating the growth and/or activity of one or a limited number of bacteria in the colon, that can improve host health".[1]

- So far, only carbohydrates have been found to be *prebiotic*, and the most effective of these are the non-digestible oligosaccharides (NDOs).

- NDOs are a form of soluble dietary fibre. They consist of sugar molecules linked together to make larger carbohydrate molecules.

- Unlike most carbohydrates (sugars and starch), NDOs are not digested in the small intestine. They work by being fermented in the colon and the terminal ileum by resident probiotic bacteria, which, as a result, increase in numbers.

- NDOs may also work by drawing harmful bacteria away from attachment to the gut wall.

- NDOs boost the numbers of bifidobacteria if those numbers are low, but not if the numbers are already high.

- People with Crohn's and severe UC appear to have low numbers of bifidobacteria and lactobacilli, and *prebiotics* may be able to raise the number of these bacteria at least temporarily.

- There is a small number of studies on the effects of *prebiotics* on inflamed intestine and these have indicated positive benefits, but more and larger studies are required.

- A drawback with NDOs is the tendency to increase gas production (flatulence and bloating). This may vary between NDOs, and the gas may be reduced if the *prebiotics* are introduced gradually.

- Compared with probiotics, NDOs are easier to store and cheaper to produce.

7. Specific *Prebiotics*

"I am 51 years old, and have been a sufferer from proctitis/ colitis for about 35 years. Although I accept that my condition is nowhere near as severe as many others, some attacks in the past have been severe and extended. About 2 years ago I came across a probiotic fruit juice with added oatmeal, and started to take a 200ml glass every day. Since that time, attacks have been very infrequent and much less severe and although I am not cured I am convinced that taking this product has been very beneficial."

This chapter looks at specific *prebiotics*, identifies their known characteristics, and shows how they might be useful for IBD.

NDOs as food

Some non-digestible oligosaccharides (NDOs) are found naturally in plants, (for example, chicory, Jerusalem artichoke, onion, leek, garlic, asparagus and banana and, to a lesser extent, in cereals). These all contain the *pre*biotic NDOs, inulin and oligofructose (FOS).

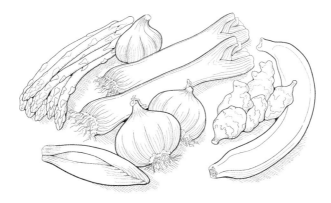

Fig 11. Asparagus, chicory, leek, onion, garlic, Jerusalem artichoke, banana

In general terms, increasing the amount of these foods in your diet will help to increase the numbers of beneficial bacteria in your lower intestines.

But how much *pre*biotic is needed to have an effect in increasing the numbers of bifidobacteria? A review of eight studies on humans, using oligofructose and inulin, showed significant increases in bifidobacterial numbers with the daily consumption of between 4 and 40 grams.[1]

Only one study used as little as 4g a day and here the increase in bifidobacterial numbers was only 14 per cent of the total increase in bacterial numbers.[2] Most studies used quantities in the range of 8-15g a day.

The only study on patients with IBD used 8.5g of an NDO per day, and resulted in 'bowel movement improvement' in four out of seven patients.[3]

How does the consumption of an extra 8g a day of NDO compare with the daily consumption of NDOs in the normal diet?

A study by the US Department of Agriculture recorded the food intake of 15,000 individuals. It was calculated that Americans consume on average 2.6g a day of oligofructose and 2.5g a day of inulin. Of this, approximately 70 per cent was obtained from wheat and 24 per cent from onions.[4]

So approximately 5g a day of food-based *pre*biotic is consumed, on average, in the American diet and about a further 8g a day of NDOs are needed to increase substantially the numbers of bifidobacteria and lactobacilli.

It does not seem very practical, for most people, to more than double the amount of wheat and onions in their daily diet for a sustainable period.

An alternative is to look at NDO products, developed from plants and sugars, that might be used as *pre*biotic supplements.

Production of NDOs

NDOs are produced by three main methods:

- by extracting them directly from a plant;
- by breaking down a polysaccharide (a longer-chain carbohydrate); or

- by binding several short-chain sugars (mono and disaccharides) together to form longer-chain carbohydrates.

Most molecules of oligosaccharides consist of between three and 10 saccharides (sugars) chemically bound together.[5] A polysaccharide molecule can consist of more than 50 chains of sugar bound together. The number of sugar molecules chained together to make a *pre*biotic may be significant for people with IBD. (See 'Targeting inflammation' later in this chapter.)

The NDOs that are best known, most researched and most readily available are:

- inulin
- fructo-oligosaccharides (FOS)
- transgalacto-oligosaccharides (TOS)
- lactulose

Inulin

Inulin has many more sugar chains per molecule than most *pre*biotics. It is usually obtained from the roots of the chicory plant, and has been produced commercially in Europe since 1920 as an industrial food ingredient. More than 70 per cent of the dried root of chicory is inulin.

The inulin is removed by soaking the chicory in hot water. The resulting product is approximately 90 per cent inulin, so there is a high level of purity. The remaining 10 per cent mostly comprises short-chain sugars.

The inulin from chicory is made up of carbohydrate with differing lengths of sugar molecule chains, ranging from three to 60 sugars per molecule, with an average of 10.[6]

There is a 'high performance' version of inulin in which the shorter molecules have been removed, and which has an average of about 25 sugar chains per molecule. This version is used for texture improvement and fat replacement in manufactured foods.[7]

Inulin is a white powder with no taste and has a low calorific value.

Inulin is undigested

A method of finding out what types of food are digested in the small intestine is to examine the faecal waste of ileostomists. A person with a permanent ileostomy is someone whose colon has been surgically removed and the end of the small intestine brought out through a stoma (an opening on the abdomen).

The waste from the small intestine is collected in a bag that is attached to the end of the intestine protruding from the stoma on the abdomen. By examining this waste it is possible to assess what part of the food has not been digested, and check what proportion of a *pre*biotic has resisted digestion in the small intestine.

Studies have shown that almost all inulin (87 per cent) survives intact after passage through stomach acid, bile salts and small intestine enzymes, to the terminal ileum (lower end of the small intestine).

Evidence of prebiotic benefit from inulin

Several studies have shown that inulin boosts the numbers of beneficial bacteria, mainly bifidobacteria, and does not increase harmful microbes such as clostridia and *E. coli*. In a study of eight subjects, Gibson and colleagues showed that the addition of 15g of oligofructose or inulin to the diet led to bifidobacteria becoming the largest bacterial group in the faeces.[8] In a further study, initiated to test the effects of lactose or inulin on bowel habits of constipated elderly patients, inulin significantly increased the numbers of bifidobacteria.[9]

Fructo-oligosaccharides (FOS)

FOS (also known as oligofructose) can be produced either by hydrolysis (breaking down) of inulin from chicory, or by linking together chains of sucrose with enzymes. The production of FOS results in a high level of purity, as there is a large proportion of the oligofructose and only a small proportion of other items such as short-chain sugars.

FOS is made up of between two and eight-sugar chain molecules, with an average of four.[7] It has a slightly sweet taste and is available as a white powder or as colourless syrup.

As a *pre*biotic, its characteristics are similar to inulin:

• low calorific value

• survives intact to the colon (approximately 90 per cent)

• boosts the number of bifidobacteria

In a review of four human studies, in which volunteers were fed a diet supplemented with between four and 12 grams a day of FOS, Roberfroid and colleagues reported that all studies "showed a significant increase in bifidobacteria in faeces".[6]

The recorded effects on other bacteria have varied in different studies, possibly because of the variability in content of different FOS products (that is, different mixtures of chain lengths of this carbohydrate).[10]

Transgalacto-oligosaccharides (TOS)

Unlike inulin and FOS, which consist of carbohydrates made up of chains of the sugar fructose, transgalacto-oligosaccharide (TOS) is made up of lactose chains. Lactose is milk sugar and is found in human breast milk. TOS, also known as galacto-oligosaccharide, is produced in commercial quantities from cows' milk, by linking the lactose molecules together with the help of enzymes.

The resulting product is not as pure as inulin or FOS. Purity is usually not more than 60 per cent, with the other ingredients consisting of the simple sugars, glucose and galactose (by-products of the enzyme action), and unused lactose.

TOS molecules range from two to eight lactose molecules in length. Mostly, however, they are three lactose molecules long.

Several studies have shown that TOS survives intact through to the lower intestine and its ingestion leads to increases in the numbers of bifidobacteria and lactobacilli.

TOS is slightly sweeter than FOS. (The longer the sugar-chain in each oligosaccharide molecule, the less sweet the product.) Like FOS, TOS is available in syrup and powder form.

Another characteristic of TOS is that it is very stable under hot and acidic conditions. Therefore, there may be potential for developing bakery products that include TOS, which would survive the high temperatures of baking, and would resist being broken down by stomach acid.

Lactulose

Lactulose is a disaccharide (a two-sugar chain carbohydrate). Unlike other *pre*biotics, it is classified as a drug rather than as a food. This is because, since the 1950s, it has been used for medical purposes, notably hepatic encephalopathy (coma caused by liver disease) and chronic constipation.

In Italy, the Netherlands and Japan, however, lactulose is classified as a food. In fact, in Japan lactulose is added to some manufactured baby foods.

Lactulose is produced from lactose, synthesised with the use of enzymes (like TOS). It has the same number of carbon, hydrogen and oxygen atoms and the same molecular weight as lactose (milk sugar), but it differs from lactose as it is not digestible. Its purity is about 80 per cent, with the remaining 20 per cent being digestible sugars.

As with most other *prebiotics*, lactulose is available either as a syrup or a powder, and has a sweet taste (about three-quarters as sweet as sucrose – table sugar).

Lactulose has been recognised as a *prebiotic* (bifidogenic) since 1957. For example, a well-designed controlled human study showed that 20g per day of lactulose over a four-week period led to a substantial increase in bifidobacteria and lactobacilli (approximately 1000-fold and 100-fold respectively). The study also showed a decrease in potentially harmful bacteria. For example, clostridia were reduced to less than one per cent of their original number.[11]

In a study referred to in Chapter 6, lactulose reduced colitis in mice, and by an equivalent amount to that of a probiotic lactobacillus[12].

In countries where lactulose is only available legally as a drug, a pharmacist or physician has to authorise its issue. Furthermore, its licensed use does not cover stimulation of probiotic bacteria for people with IBD.

Lactitol is similar to lactulose. It is a disaccharide (two-sugar chain molecule) produced from lactose, and is used as a drug for the same purposes as lactulose. It acts as a *prebiotic*, but the evidence suggests that it is less effective than lactulose.

Other *prebiotics*

In addition to the 'big four' *prebiotics* there are others that are more recent developments emanating from Japan. These are:

- Isomalto-oligosaccharides (ISO) – from starch
- Soyo-oligosaccharides (SOS) – from soya beans

- Xylo-oligosaccharides (XOS) – from corn cobs
- Lactosucrose (LS) – a synthesis of sucrose and lactose

All the above are used in foods in Japan, particularly in soft drinks and as tabletop sweeteners. There are very few studies on how they may alter the bacterial flora in humans, although limited evidence points to bifidobacteria being increased.

An additional difficulty in assessing research evidence is that the purity of some of these products is poor. One study found that the XOS came with large quantities of starch and some simple sugars. The proportion of xylo-oligosaccharide by weight was only 34 per cent.[1]

These newer *prebiotics* do include lactosucrose which was used in the only study of a *prebiotic* on people with IBD (see chapter 6). The results were encouraging.

Other *prebiotics* for which there is even less evidence are: gluco-oligosaccharides, including polydextrose (synthesised from glucose); palatinose (synthesised from sucrose); and pyrodextrin (from maize or potato starch).

Other carbohydrates are being considered as *prebiotics*, such as resistant starch, and acacia gum (gum arabic), but information is very limited.[13]

Comparing the *prebiotics*

One laboratory-based study has compared seven NDO *prebiotics*. The main findings were:

- All prebiotics increased bifidobacteria and most decreased clostridia.
- Xylo-oligosaccharides and lactulose produced the highest increases in bifidobacteria.
- FOS produced the highest populations of lactobacilli.
- GOS resulted in the largest decreases in clostridia.
- Short-chain fatty acid generation was highest with lactulose and GOS.
- Gas production was lowest with isomalto-oligosaccharides and highest with inulin.

It should be noted, however, that laboratory-based studies (known as *in vitro*) can only give a limited picture. The bacterial interactions in the human intestine are so complex that comparisons will have to be undertaken in human trials to provide a reasonable picture of the differing effects of the individual *pre*biotics.[14] So far, however, there has been almost no comparison of *pre*biotics in human studies.

Genus, species, or strain

One significant weakness in research on the effects of *pre*biotics is that studies have only measured the changes in the gut flora at the genus (family) level, rather than at the species level.

It is known that the behaviour of bacteria varies considerably according to species, and may vary between strains where there are tiny differences between members of the same species.

A. J. McBain and G. T. Macfarlane have stated that "it is simplistic to assume that all species or strains of bifidobacteria and lactobacilli have probiotic properties and, in any case, these will be highly variable".[15]

Until changes caused by *pre*biotics are measured in greater detail, it is difficult to know precisely the effect of specific *pre*biotics on the gut microflora.

New and robust molecular techniques of identifying bacteria are, however, being developed.

Targeting inflammation

Despite the large numbers of unknowns, it is nevertheless possible to state that an increase in the number of bifidobacteria and lactobacilli is likely to have beneficial effects. Does one type of *pre*biotic work better than others on a particular part of the intestine?

To answer this question, a theory is set out below. Please note, however, that there is no evidence recorded in human studies to support or reject the theory.

The key issue in targeting IBD with *pre*biotics may be the number of sugars that are linked together to form one NDO molecule. The more sugar molecules that form an NDO molecule, the longer it takes for bacteria to break it down. For example, laboratory experiments have shown that, NDOs with a chain length of greater than 10 sugars, are fermented on average half as quickly as molecules consisting of less than 10 sugars.[6]

Gibson and his colleagues commented that "it is reasonable to assume that the longer the oligosaccharides, the further the *pre*biotic effect may penetrate the colon".[16] In support of this, a study on rats with colitis found an increasing acidity in the distal colon when inulin was added to the diet. This suggests that some of the inulin (10-sugar molecules on average) was reaching the lower part of the colon and stimulating acid-producing beneficial bacteria.[17] In comparison, FOS (four-sugar molecules on average) is known to be completely fermented before reaching the distal colon.

Therefore, if IBD affects the lower end of the colon, inulin might be the preferred *pre*biotic. This is because it has long chains of sugars that make up its molecules. NDOs with short-chain molecules may be more suitable for inflammation in the ileum and proximal (upper) colon.

Synbiotics

Synbiotics is the term used for the combination of probiotics and *pre*biotics.

Gibson and Roberfroid defined synbiotics as "a mixture of probiotics and *pre*biotics that beneficially affects the host by improving the survival and implantation of live microbial dietary supplements in the gastrointestinal tract, by selectively stimulating the growth and/or by activating the metabolism of one or a limited number of health-promoting bacteria, and thus improving host welfare".[18]

The synbiotic combination has three potential benefits. The *pre*biotic may physically protect bacteria from injury or death as a result of stomach acid and other intestinal chemicals, as well as providing a food while it passes down the gut.

Secondly, the *pre*biotic may help the probiotic to become implanted in the terminal ileum or colon, by keeping other bacteria from attachment sites, and by aiding the probiotic bacteria to be in good condition.

Thirdly, the *pre*biotic may stimulate the growth and activity of the probiotic while it lives in the slow-moving lower gut. It may also stimulate health-promoting bifidobacteria and lactobacilli that are already part of the gut flora.

The idea of combining probiotics and *pre*biotics is therefore attractive, but at the moment there is very little evidence in human studies relating to the effects of such mixtures.

Chapter summary

- There are four main NDOs that have *pre*biotic effects: inulin, fructo-oligosaccharides (FOS), transgalacto-oligosaccharides (TOS) and lactulose.

- Inulin and FOS can be obtained from the chicory plant. Several other plants contain significant amounts of inulin and FOS.

- Unlike other NDOs that are classified as food or food supplements, lactulose is classified as a drug in most countries. Otherwise, it is not significantly different from the other NDOs.

- There are other NDOs, but almost no research has been undertaken on their potential *pre*biotic effects on humans.

- A weakness of research into *pre*biotics is that only genus numbers are being taken into account rather than specific species. New molecular measures of identifying bacteria will help to resolve this problem.

- In theory, NDOs with short chain molecules may be more quickly fermented and therefore benefit the terminal ileum and the proximal (upper) colon. The long chain NDOs may take longer to be fermented and some may have an effect in the distal (lower) colon.

- Synbiotics is the combining of probiotics and *pre*biotics to maximise the effects of both.

8. Other Benefits of Probiotics

"After a severe attack of diarrhoea which put me in hospital, my doctor prescribed an antibiotic for five days, followed by a good yoghurt. The idea was to kill harmful bacteria that were causing excessive flatus and replace these with the bifidobacteria in the yoghurt. The flatulence changed to normal within twenty-four hours. I have been taking the yoghurt for nine months, 75g twice a day, with no drugs. The diarrhoea and flatus associated with my Crohn's is almost non existent so far."

This chapter considers what evidence there is for probiotics helping intestinal conditions, which may also affect people with IBD. The conditions covered are:

- Non-IBD diarrhoea
- Constipation
- Cancer of the colon
- Irritable Bowel Syndrome (IBS)
- Lactose intolerance

Non-IBD diarrhoea

Diarrhoea is the excessive loss of water from the gastrointestinal tract. In addition to being a major symptom of IBD, it can also be the result of activity by infectious microbes or as a consequence of taking antibiotics.

Gastroenteritis (infectious diarrhoea)

Gastroenteritis is the main cause of acute diarrhoea.[1] It is caused by toxins from harmful microbes that trigger copious secretions from the intestine wall, aimed at flushing away the harmful agents.

Although in some cases the cause of infectious diarrhoea may be serious (for example, amoebic dysentery, typhoid, cholera), in most cases the causal agent is less serious. Diarrhoea usually ends after two or three days without active treatment. People with IBD may, however, experience relapses of UC or Crohn's after a diarrhoeal infection.

The evidence for probiotics preventing infectious diarrhoea is not clear-cut, possibly because the number of different pathogens that may be responsible for this type of diarrhoea is very large, and because it is likely that not all probiotics will work against all pathogens.

Current evidence indicates that probiotics help to:

- reduce the incidence of some types of 'traveller's diarrhoea';[2]
- reduce the incidence among children of diarrhoea acquired while resident in hospital;[3]
- shorten the time of recovery, particularly in diarrhoea caused by rotavirus; and
- improve chronic diarrhoea caused by the HIV virus.[4]

Antibiotic-associated diarrhoea (AAD)

In approximately 20 per cent of patients receiving antibiotic treatment, diarrhoea will develop.[2] Antibiotic treatment may result in "a severe attack on the normal gastrointestinal flora"[5] and in the resulting 'vacuum', harmful microbes may become established.

AAD is of particular relevance to people with Crohn's, as antibiotics are a recognised form of treatment. Pathogenic bacteria may be causing additional problems in Crohn's because of the narrowing of the bore of the small intestine as a result of ulceration. Food can back up behind the constriction, waiting to move slowly through the narrowed area. This relatively static food may encourage an overgrowth of bacteria, some of which may be harmful.

But the use of antibiotics to eliminate the overgrowth of harmful bacteria may also decimate the microflora. The 'barrier effect' exerted by the normal microflora against the colonisation of newly arrived microbes is weakened and new pathogens can become established.

Several randomised controlled trials, involving more than eight hundred patients, have been undertaken to see whether the use of probiotics will reduce the risk of diarrhoea developing in those taking antibiotics. The results have been positive, with several products (most containing *Saccharomyces boulardii* or lactobacilli) providing a significant reduction in risk. On average, about half the number of patients developed diarrhoea compared with those not taking the probiotic. Rial Rolfe concluded that "patients at risk of developing antibiotic-associated diarrhoea would benefit from prophylactic probiotic therapy".[2]

*Pre*biotics may also help. A study on mice, in which antibiotic use led to salmonella infection, showed a reduction in infection through the administration of some strains of bifidobacteria. The probiotic effect improved with the addition of a *pre*biotic.[6]

Persistent Clostridium difficile

One of the most common pathogens to fill the vacuum created by antibiotics is *Clostridium difficile*. The diarrhoea that it causes is a type of infectious diarrhoea.

Antibiotics treat the *Clostridium difficile* infection, but this pathogen can be very persistent, sometimes forming spores and surviving in the intestine. It can therefore recur, and does so in approximately 20 per cent of patients who have been treated on one occasion with antibiotics. Of those with several episodes of *C. difficile* disease, 40 per cent will have a recurrence after antibiotic treatment.[1]

Some limited probiotic studies have been undertaken on patients with active *C. difficile* disease, with encouraging signs of reduced infection. More research is needed, however, to confirm that probiotics are effective against this persistent bacterium.

Constipation

With diarrhoea there is too much water and fluid in the faeces, but with constipation (the infrequent passing of stools) there is too little. Constipation may be a symptom of IBD and there are two main reasons why it may appear.

The intestinal tube may narrow as a result of ulceration arising from IBD inflammation, slowing the passage of undigested food. Also, some people with IBD (particularly Crohn's) may be advised to eat a low-fibre diet to avoid aggravating the inflamed lining of the intestine.

If food is moving slowly in the intestine and/or is lacking fibre, too much water may be removed along with the nutrients during the digestion process. The faeces become hard and constipation occurs.

In a review of fourteen studies, despite caution about some of the methodologies and difficulties in comparing like with like, the conclusion was that "the effect of probiotics on gut transit times and stool frequency is probable".[7]

*Pre*biotics are known to have an effect in reducing constipation. This is not surprising as they are a type of soluble fibre. For example, a study using the*pre*biotic long-chain inulin (15g per day) on healthy volunteers with low stool frequency (one stool every two to three days), found a "significant increase in stool frequency"[8].

Cancer of the colon

Colon cancer is a major cause of death in older people in the western world. Each year in the United States, 50-60,000 people die from this form of cancer and 130-160,000 new cases are diagnosed.

The exact cause of the disease is not known. Some known risk factors are:

- age over 50
- a family history of colonic cancer
- a high fat, low fibre diet
- a sedentary life
- longstanding and extensive UC, and prolonged and severe Crohn's of the colon[9].

Because of the nature of cancer, it has been difficult to devise probiotic experiments on humans, but there have been plenty of studies on mice and rats. These experimental studies suggest a probiotic effect of improving colon cancer protection[10].

In particular, there is evidence that yoghurt and some fermented milks may reduce cancer[11]. Laboratory studies have indicated that chemical products of the fermentation process by yoghurt bacteria are effective in deactivating cancer-causing chemicals[12].

A review that considered all studies undertaken over the previous 10 years concluded that "there appears to be a synergistic effect of consumption of probiotic bacteria and *pre*biotics such as fructo-oligosaccharides on the attenuation [reduction] of the development of colon cancer. The effect is often not large, but it is possible it could be beneficial, in combination with other ways to reduce risk".[13]

Studies of the use of *prebiotics* alone have also shown anti-cancer benefits. For example, a recent study showed that oligofructose and inulin reduced the number of precancerous cells in the colon of mice.[14]

A review of research on *prebiotics* and colon cancer in mice and rats indicated that inulin provided a greater benefit than oligofructose. As colon cancer occurs more often in the distal (lower) rather than the proximal (upper) colon, the greater benefit of inulin may be because of "the lower fermentation rate of the inulin, which as a consequence may arrive in more distal parts of the colon".[15] Inulin has larger molecules and it takes longer for the bacteria to break them down. Therefore not all of the inulin has been fermented by the time it reaches the last part of the colon.

Another interesting discovery, using animal models, is that the use of inulin and oligofructose in conjunction with anti-cancer drugs increases the effectiveness of the drugs. There seems to be a synergistic effect, whereby the benefit is greater than might be expected from adding two treatments together.[16]

Why might probiotics and prebiotics help?

Some bacteria in the normal microflora produce enzymes that might be a factor in increased cancer risk. An increased proportion of probiotic bacteria in the microflora may reduce that effect. As Ross Crittenden explains, "Bifidobacteria and lactic acid bacteria have low activities of these enzymes compared to other major anaerobes in the gut such as bacteroides, eubacteria, and clostridia".[17] [Anaerobes are bacteria that live without oxygen, and the colon has virtually no oxygen in it].

Also, some bacteria in the normal microflora convert bile acids into forms that may promote cancer. Probiotic bacteria may increase acidity in the colon, however, and so reduce the numbers of those bacteria that break down the bile acids.

Irritable bowel syndrome (IBS)

IBS is the most common condition considered by hospital gastroenterology clinics and it has been diagnosed in 2.9 per cent of the US population.[18] Its cause is not known. No damage is done to the intestine, but the colon does not seem to be working properly, in that muscle contractions are irregular and more sensitive to stimulation.

The main symptoms are abdominal pain, and diarrhoea or constipation. There may also be bloating and flatulence. Sometimes IBS starts after infectious diarrhoea or antibiotic use. Stress and food intolerances are also associated with this condition.

People with IBD can also have IBS. Although it may be difficult to separate out some of the symptoms, there is no evidence of a connection between the two conditions.

IBS is diagnosed by ruling out alternative explanations of the symptoms and, as such, it may be a term covering several similar conditions rather than just one.

As it is a fluctuating condition, and the placebo effect may be high (where patients think themselves better even though they are receiving only a blank treatment), it is especially important to look at randomised controlled trials (RCTs) when examining the results of treatment with probiotics.

In a review of five RCTs, improvement in health was experienced by between 30 and 61 per cent of those who had received the placebo. Despite this high level of placebo-response, however, these five studies, involving a total of 720 patients "showed a statistically significant outcome benefit from taking probiotics".[19]

A more recent study has also given encouraging results. Using *Lactobacillus plantarum* 299v, 19 out of 20 patients receiving the probiotic showed improvement in all IBS symptoms compared with three out of 20 in the placebo group.[20]

As there have also been some negative results, however, one reviewer concluded that the level of evidence that probiotics help people with IBS is very low.[3]

Lactose intolerance

The term 'lactose intolerance' refers to the inability of some adults to digest the sugar lactose, which is present in milk. Lactose is digested by the enzyme lac*tase* (written here with an italicised suffix to distinguish it). Those with lactose intolerance produce too little lac*tase* to digest much of the milk sugar, and the undigested lactose causes intestinal difficulties.

8: Other Benefits of Probiotics

Most of the world's adult population are lactose intolerant. For them, "lact*ase* activity is high at birth, decreases in childhood and adolescence, and remains low in adulthood".[21] Those with low lact*ase* levels may be able to digest small amounts of milk. Studies suggest that most people who are lactose intolerant can tolerate 12.5-25g of milk a day without significant symptoms developing.[22]

When people with lactose intolerance consume milk they may suffer from excess gas, bloating, diarrhoea, cramps, abdominal rumblings and flatulence, with occasional nausea and vomiting in severe cases.

The excess gas is probably caused by the gut microflora fermenting the lactose. The diarrhoea may be caused by an osmotic response to the lactose, leading to high water content in the faeces being maintained.

There may be an additional problem for some people with Crohn's. Lactose is mostly digested in the upper part of the small intestine (the jejunum). If the small intestine is inflamed, it is less effective in producing enzymes, including lact*ase*. Therefore, if a person's Crohn's inflammation is present in the jejunum, more milk may be undigested leading to lactose intolerance.

Yoghurt benefits

The probiotic product yoghurt is particularly helpful in reducing the symptoms of lactose intolerance. Numerous studies have shown better lactose digestion and less flatulence in lactose-intolerant people who consumed nonheated yoghurt rather than milk or pasteurised yoghurt.[21]

One study reported a 66 per cent improvement in lactose digestion using yoghurt rather than milk.[23]

The yoghurt bacteria (*L. bulgaricus* and *S. thermophilus*) produce significant quantities of their own lact*ase* enzyme, by which they are able to digest lactose in the live yoghurt. Fermentation continues as the yoghurt is eaten, further reducing lactose and producing less gas than other bacteria. Diarrhoea is reduced or eliminated.

Yoghurt also slows down the rate at which milk passes through the intestine, allowing more time for lact*ase* to digest the lactose. It is likely that yoghurt takes longer than milk to travel through the intestine because of its thicker consistency.

There is limited evidence that the Russian fermented milk *kefir* is also effective in reducing lactose intolerance.[24] Studies on a range of other fermented milks (containing different bacteria) showed significantly less effect in digesting lactose.[25] Thus not all fermented milks have the same characteristics.

Other probiotics

Probiotic products in capsule, tablet or powder form (for example, lactobacillus and bifidobacterium species used in non-milk products) do not appear to be as effective as yoghurt in alleviating lactose intolerance.

The bacterial enzyme that breaks down lactose is rendered inactive in very acidic conditions. The milk in yoghurt may act as a buffer, protecting the bacteria from stomach acid.

*Pre*biotics should be able to increase the number of lactobacilli in the microflora, which in turn should increase the digestion of lactose without the development of excess gas.

One small study has supported this theory. Nine people with lactose intolerance received 10g of lactulose twice daily for a three-week period. Eight had improved symptoms, including three who had improved so much they no longer met the criteria for lactose intolerance.[26]

Chapter summary

- Probiotics have been shown to reduce the likelihood of developing gastroenteritis and to accelerate the recovery time.

- Various lactic acid producing bacteria as well as *Saccharomyces boulardii* have been shown to reduce the risk of developing antibiotic-associated diarrhoea.

- Probiotics may help to eradicate recurring *Clostridium difficile* infection.

- There is limited evidence that some probiotics may relieve constipation; however the evidence for *pre*biotics alleviating constipation is much stronger.

- Animal studies and laboratory tests suggest that yoghurt and some other fermented milks may help to reduce the risk of colon cancer. *Pre*biotics, particularly those with long-chain molecules, may also be beneficial.

- The evidence for probiotics relieving irritable bowel syndrome is weak, although this may in part be due to the wide variability of the condition.

- Yoghurt and *kefir* have been shown to reduce lactose intolerance. *Pre*biotics may also help.

9. Questions & Answers on Probiotics

"I have UC of 23 years standing. I cannot take steroid tablets and the other drugs have brought me out in hives. I found some relief when I eliminated the cabbage family out of my diet and then discovered non-milk probiotics in Finland, which made a big difference. I gradually introduced the milky probiotics, as my calcium levels were falling. After 6 months I find I only need a dose of probiotic once or twice a week. I have settled into a fairly regular pattern of formed stools, after all these years, and I am feeling a lot better than I have for a long time."

This final chapter uses the format of questions and answers to reiterate the main points in the book, to discuss practical matters, and to consider what the future may hold.

Q. Are probiotics a cure for IBD?

A. Currently, there is no known cure for IBD. Probiotics have been shown to alleviate symptoms in some clinical studies, but it is not yet clear how effective they are. If probiotics become part of conventional treatment, it will most probably be in combination with other medication that help to combat these complex diseases.

Q. Should I consider taking them?

A. Probiotics are unusual in that they are a treatment at an early stage of clinical investigation for IBD, and yet are already widely available. The decision you take is one that involves your medical history and current medication. Any time, therefore, that you consider taking something to affect IBD it is advised that a discussion with your doctor be the first step.

If your doctor is reluctant to consider probiotics, the reasons may include the following:

- The medical profession concentrates on diagnosis and treatment. Treatment is intended to change the health of the patient in a planned and logical way, drawing on the existing knowledge of medical science. So far, most gastroenterologists have not been convinced that beneficial bacteria can be used in a reliable and predictable way to benefit people with IBD.
- Probiotic products are classified as food or food supplements in most countries, and doctors do not usually prescribe food as treatment for disease.

Despite these difficulties it is still better to try to involve your doctor in discussing the probiotic option.

Q. What makes a good probiotic product?

A. Here is a list of some likely desirable elements:

- A large number of bacteria in each dose (many products contain between one and five billion bacteria);
- The probiotic should be packaged and stored so that there is only a small reduction in numbers of live bacteria from the time of production to the time of sale;
- Protection from the effects of stomach acid; for example, enteric coating, inclusion with milk or fruit juice, or by using acid-resistant strains of bacteria;
- Food to enable the bacteria to live and grow as they travel through the intestine. This is usually supernatant (remains of the food in which the bacteria were originally grown), or non-digestible carbohydrate;
- Species and strains that can colonise the human gut, at least temporarily;
- Species and strains for which there is some scientific evidence of health benefit;
- A mixture of probiotic species, rather than only one species, to increase the chances that at least one will be very effective.

Q. How easy is it to find this information?

A. Unfortunately, much of this information is unavailable on the packaging and literature of probiotic products. For example, most probiotic foods do not state how many bacteria they contain. And with probiotic supplements, some may state the number of bacteria at the time of manufacture, but few guarantee the minimum number that remain alive after a specified time.

In general terms, the more information that a company provides the more likely it is to be producing a sound and substantial product. On the other hand, if the product description is strong on emotional language and weak on facts you might be more sceptical of what it really has to offer.

Q. Can I trust what the manufacturer says about the probiotic product?

A. Unfortunately not always. Since the 1970s a number of analyses of probiotic products have shown a poor correlation between the claimed and actual content.[1]

More recently, a detailed examination of 52 probiotic products available in the UK and continental Europe found that:

- None of the bio-yoghurts stated how many bacteria they contained.
- Three products did not have any live bacteria, and nine products had fewer than 10 per cent of the numbers of bacteria claimed.
- Many products contained different bacteria to those stated on the label.[2]

Q. What are the particular strengths of a milk-based probiotic?

A. Milk-based probiotics, which are classified as food, have the advantage that the bacteria are more protected from the effects of stomach acid. This is important as stomach acid kills a large proportion (often more than 90 per cent) of 'unprotected' bacteria. Milk acts as a buffer against the acid.[3]

Fermentation in milk can produce added benefits. Some products, notably 'acidophilus milk', use unfermented milk with added probiotic bacteria, but most milk-based probiotics have been fermented by the bacteria they contain.

The most common type of fermented milk in the Western world is yoghurt. The two types of bacteria that are used to produce yoghurt do not stay long in the human intestine before being passed out as part of the stools. The by-products of the fermentation of yoghurt bacteria, which remain a part of the yoghurt, are, however, known to provide health benefits.

Q. What are the strengths of non-milk probiotics?

A. Non-milk probiotics, which are usually classified as food supplements, come in a range of forms, including powders, tablets and capsules. Many of these products give a figure of the numbers of bacteria contained at the time of manufacture. In comparison, it is rare for milk-based probiotic foods to quantify their bacterial contents.

The probiotic supplements usually have a long shelf-life, much longer than milk-based probiotics. This is because most supplements are freeze-dried. This is a process whereby the growth medium containing the bacteria is first frozen and then the water is removed to the point that the bacteria remain alive but inactive. When water is added they become active again.

If the freeze-drying is done well, then the probiotic supplement can be stored safely at room temperature. This does not happen in all cases, and it can be a difficult process if very large concentrations of bacteria are being freeze-dried. Some freeze-dried probiotics may therefore need to be kept in a refrigerator.

Q. Where can I obtain probiotics?

A. Milk-based probiotics can be found in supermarkets, while probiotic supplements are available from health food stores and from mail-order vitamin, mineral and herbal remedy companies.

Q. Where can I obtain *prebiotics*?

A. As with probiotic supplements, *prebiotics*, in the form of powdered supplements can be obtained from health food stores and mail-order companies. The two most commonly available *prebiotics* are FOS (oligofructose) and inulin. Some probiotic foods also contain added *pre*biotics.

Q. Can a *pre*biotic add to the effects of probiotic bacteria?

A. *Pre*biotics are food for probiotic bacteria. Bifidobacteria and, to a lesser extent, lactobacilli, find *pre*biotics easier to ferment than do other less desirable bacteria. Research has shown that taking *pre*biotics increases the numbers of beneficial bacteria in the microflora, and provides food for the probiotics you are consuming.

Q. If a probiotic helps to relieve the severity of IBD, why doesn't it work permanently?

A. One of the reasons why there are vast numbers of bacteria resident in the human intestine is that they act as a defence against harmful invading microbes. The various types of resident bacteria colonise different parts of the intestine by attaching themselves to the gut wall or by growing on the partly digested food in the more slowly moving parts of the intestine. By occupying these best positions in the gut they make it difficult for invading bacteria to become established.

This process is known as 'colonisation resistance' and it works against all newly arrived bacteria, including probiotics. This is probably why probiotic bacteria do not become established permanently.

Q. How do genetics influence the microflora?

A. A study of five pairs of identical and five pairs of non-identical twins, showed that the intestinal flora were very similar in the identical twins, but much less so with the non-identical twins.[4] This suggests that genetic influence over a person's usual gut microflora is substantial.

In some individuals the microflora may have a greater tendency to change than in other individuals. In a year-long study, the strains of lactobacilli and bifidobacteria in two people were monitored closely. In one subject there were five strains of bifidobacteria present for the whole year. The other person had a changing population of different bifidobacteria strains.

Theoretically, the microfloral pattern of the latter might be more prone to being influenced by probiotic bacteria.[5]

Q. Will taking probiotics and *prebiotics* regularly change the gut microflora so that it becomes properly balanced?

A. Many probiotic products claim that they promote a 'healthy balance' of bacteria in the intestine, but it is not clear what an ideal balance is, or even if there is such an ideal state.

It is known, however, that there is a shortage of lactic acid bacteria in people with IBD and it is also known that the gut microflora play an important part in continuing the IBD inflammation, and possibly in starting it. Therefore, although what comprises a proper balance is not yet known, increasing the numbers of lactobacilli and bifidobacteria may help people with IBD.

Microscopic examination of human faecal content has revealed approximately 400 bacterial species, but only about two-thirds of these have been identified. Of those identified, about 30-40 species make up 99 per cent of the total population of gut bacteria in any one individual.[6]

New molecular techniques of assessing bacterial strains through genetic material have been introduced.[7] This will allow a much better picture to develop of the species and strains present in healthy populations; and this, in turn, will allow more planned corrections of the abnormal microflora of people with intestinal disorders, including IBD.

Q. Can probiotics be used with children?

A. There are no published studies of probiotics used in children with IBD, although probiotics have been used effectively in children against infectious diarrhoea.[8] There is a lot of interest in the potential of probiotics for children with IBD because, if they are shown to be effective, it should mean that the amount of prescribed drugs could be reduced and surgery might be avoided.

In infants, caution should be shown, as their immune system is not fully developed and the gut microflora is still becoming established. With older children, the same caution as with adults is needed. If immuno-suppressant drugs are being taken, care is needed in case those with lowered immune systems are more vulnerable to opportunistic infections.

Q. Are researchers investigating ways to make probiotics available to patients with severely weakened immune systems?

A. A study involving 73 young children with acute diarrhoea found that those who received a probiotic containing killed *L. acidophilus* LB recovered more quickly compared to those of a control group.[9]

The advantage of this particular product is that there is no risk of the probiotic bacteria acting pathogenically, because the bacteria are dead. It is not yet clear how dead probiotic bacteria can still exert a beneficial effect, or how this effect compares with the same bacterium in a live state. There is, however, potential for further research on this approach.

Q. What does the future hold for probiotics and IBD?

A. There are several possibilities:

- The discovery of particular genes associated with UC and Crohn's may enable the selection for research of participants with similar disease characteristics. The research results are likely to be more reliable as a consequence.

- Increased competition between food companies and other probiotic providers is likely to lead to improved information for the customer. This could include details of the numbers of bacteria contained and the particular strengths of individual strains, including resistance to stomach acid.

- Some probiotics may become classified as drugs, or given a similar legal position. With the associated guidance that must be provided with drug status, it will be easier for physicians to prescribe the products. Also, food companies may be allowed to make health claims for some of their probiotic products, which will make the benefits of the ingredients clearer to customers.

Appendix 1:
The Body's Defence Systems

"After my Crohn's had been brought under control in hospital, I started taking natural live yoghurt. Thirteen years later I am still in remission, with no recurrences and continuing to use various makes of yoghurt, including those with bifidus bacteria. When on holiday, the hotel or supermarket will usually provide natural yoghurt. In Turkey, I automatically drank the local mix of yoghurt, salt and water which was a normal lunchtime drink for the locals."

The three main methods by which the human body defends itself from attack by pathogens (harmful agents) are:

- physical barriers
- the innate immune system
- the adaptive immune system

Physical barriers

The physical barriers stop the great majority of harmful organisms from entering the body and becoming established. These barriers are as follows:

- skin
- mucus
- gastric acid
- peristalsis

The skin is a physical barrier that protects the body from harmful microbes (bacteria, viruses, fungi) and other harmful elements (chemicals, parasites). It comprises a thick layer of cells that protects the body.

Another barrier is the mucus membrane which lines the digestive, respiratory and reproductive tracts. Mucus is a sticky substance that appears, for instance, on the inside of the nose. It collects microbes when you breathe in air, and is produced in large quantities during a cold to flush out the virus.

Skin over the body covers about two square metres, while the mucus membranes, on the inner linings of the lungs, intestine, nose and vagina, cover about 400 square metres. Of the parts of the body covered by mucus, the small intestine constitutes a large proportion because of the many tiny folds, or villi, on its surface.

Stomach acid provides another physical barrier. A very high proportion of pathogens are killed or weakened when they pass through the stomach.

Peristalsis (muscle contractions) of the intestine moves food onwards and makes it difficult for microbes to stay long enough in the intestine to become established and reproduce.

The intestine plays a significant part in the body's physical defences and it is important that it functions well. The intestine is more complex than the skin, because it has to both absorb digested food and keep out harmful agents.

Although the body's physical barriers exclude or remove the great majority of the pathogens, inevitably some will get through into the blood system, because there are such a large number of microbes.

Once pathogens enter the blood stream, the immune system starts to act.

What is the immune system?
The immune system is very complex, and scientific understanding of it is still developing. It is called a system because it involves a number of different interrelated elements. Its purpose is to defend the body from pathogens, and it consists of two elements, the innate and the adaptive.

The innate immune system
The innate system, also known as the 'non-specific' system, consists mostly of various types of white blood cells. It can act very quickly against a small number of the most common invaders.

One type of these white blood cells is known as a phagocyte, which engulfs and destroys bacteria and other foreign particles. Phagocytes were first identified by Elie Metchnikoff (see Chapter 2).

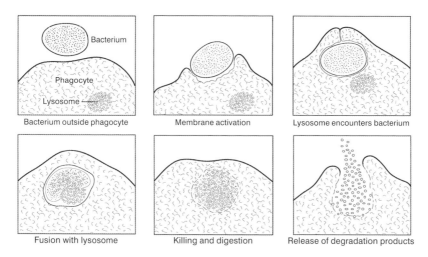

Fig 12. *Phagocyte engulfing a pathogen*

When they destroy the bacteria, the phagocytes release chemicals that affect the blood vessels and local tissues. There is a build-up of blood that causes affected areas to swell and turn red. Thus inflammation develops.

The fluid-filled swelling makes it easier for other phagocytes to reach the site of infection, together with a range of other cells and proteins that form part of the attack on the invading pathogens.

In addition to helping to develop inflammation, immune cells also produce a type of protein called a cytokine. Cytokines encourage other white blood cells that attack pathogens to reach the invasion site and so accelerate the inflammation.

One of the most recent pharmaceutical developments in treating Crohn's Disease is infliximab (Remicade®, Centocor, Inc., Malvern, PA), which neutralises the cytokine TNF-alpha.

When a large number of white blood cells gather at the site of the inflammation, pus is created. People with IBD sometimes see pus in their stools, as well as blood and mucus.

The innate immune system, in addition to being a quick and relatively simple method of attacking harmful invaders, also plays an essential role in ensuring that the more complicated adaptive immune system works.

The adaptive immune system

The system is called adaptive because the cells and proteins that are produced to attack the invading microbes differ according to the particular variety of invader.

While the innate system can deal with most common types of pathogen, the adaptive system can deal with unusual and rare pathogens. But it is slower to get going, and needs the innate system to help identify the pathogens.

One factor in the development of the adaptive system may have been viruses. Viruses are tiny one-cell creatures that grow and reproduce only within other cells. Viruses mutate (change) more readily than bacteria and thus can be dealt with rather better by the adaptive rather than the innate system.

Antibodies and antigens

An essential element in the adaptive system is the B cell, a type of white blood cell. B cells produce proteins known as antibodies. Antibodies attack invaders, the antigens. Antibodies attach themselves to the antigens, which makes it easier for phagocytes to identify and destroy them. It is an extraordinary system, because it has been calculated that there could be as many as 100 million different antigens and the adaptive system produces a different antibody for each one.

The lymph system

Certain white blood cells, B cells and T cells, travel in both the bloodstream and the lymph system.

The lymph system is a part of the immune system. It is a collection of vessels into which fluid (lymph) drains from the tissues, including the intestine. The lymph fluid is pushed through the lymph vessels in the body towards the neck, where the fluid rejoins the blood. It is often in lymph nodes (swellings) that the B and T cells first identify new pathogens.

Memory cells

Once the antigen has been destroyed, most of the B and T cells die. Enough of them remain, however, to respond to the same antigens if they reappear. If they do invade again, the remaining B and T cells (now known as memory cells) will go into action and produce masses of antibodies much more quickly than at the time of the original invasion.

This is how people are 'immunised' (protected) against an antigen once it has initially been defeated by the adaptive immune system. Vaccination against contagious diseases triggers the adaptive response to weakened versions of a virus or bacterium, so that memory cells are created to deal with the full-blown disease should it occur.

Conclusion

The body's physical barriers stop most harmful microbes from entering the bloodstream. The innate and adaptive immune systems operate together as a highly sophisticated collection of white blood cells, lymph vessels and tissue, antibody proteins and various inflammatory chemicals to defeat pathogens that manage to enter the body systems.

Appendix 2:
Safety of Probiotics

"I have suffered on and off with UC for about 18 years. When I have a flare-up it usually hospitalises me for a couple of weeks until the steroids kick in. One of the early signs that all is not right is an excessive amount of wind. I tried a probiotic milk drink and within twenty-four hours the wind and discomfort disappeared. I kept on with the probiotic for one week and then stopped. I now find that at approximately monthly intervals the wind symptoms return and I take another week's supply of the probiotic drink and it disappears again. I have been free from flare-ups for over a year now. I had a routine colonoscopy two weeks ago and the consultant said, 'Whatever you are doing keep doing it because everything looks fine'."

There are no major side effects from taking probiotics, unlike with many of the prescribed drugs for IBD. We should, however, consider what risk does exist, and under what circumstances risk is greatest.

The normal microflora

As probiotics are added to the existing gut bacteria, it is worth considering whether there are any risks from the normal microflora.

A leading bacteriologist has described the normal microflora as "a considerable hazard to the well-being of the human host".[1] The reason for this somewhat dramatic statement is that many species in the intestine are 'opportunistic pathogens'. In other words, they are normally harmless, but in some situations (for example, surgery, wounds through accident, or a severely weakened immune system) they can become virulent and cause disease.

Nevertheless, the species that comprise most probiotics are among the safest of the gut bacteria. Therefore, if anything, consumption of probiotics is likely to reduce the risk of disease arising from the microflora because the proportion of the safer bacteria will have been increased.

External bacteria and other microbes are potentially more dangerous to health, because among them will be pathogens that readily cause disease (for example, Salmonella food poisoning).

Is a discussion of risk relevant to IBD?

A discussion of risk is relevant to IBD because the drugs prescribed for UC and Crohn's are mostly aimed at dampening the immune response.

Because of this deliberate 'weakening' of the immune process, and because there may be open sores on the intestinal wall arising from inflammation, there is an increased risk of infection from both the gut microflora and invading pathogens.

This is why antibiotics are occasionally prescribed in IBD.

How much risk do probiotic products carry?

Most probiotic products contain 'human bacteria', in that they were first found in humans. As such, they do not come within the category of 'invading aliens', and therefore are less likely to be a danger.

Also, no bacteria from a probiotic product have yet been able to establish themselves in the human gut for a long period. They pass through the intestines and exert their effect, but do not form long-term reproducing colonies. Because they do not become established, the likelihood of the strains of consumed probiotics causing disease opportunistically is very low.

The following information covers risks associated with specific probiotic species and strains.

Escherichia coli Nissle 1917 ('Mutaflor')

Ardeypharm (Herdecke, Germany), the manufacturer of Mutaflor®, report one incidence of adverse effects in infants that were "seriously nutritionally disturbed" and suffering from intestinal infections. Their condition worsened.[2]

Since the introduction of reduced doses of the probiotic, however, there have been no reports of any significant side effects, and the product has subsequently been used successfully in infants.

Pathogenic strains of E. coli

Could there be any mix-up between the probiotic strain of *E. coli* and the various pathogenic strains?

The literature available from Ardeypharm states that it uses four different methods to check that the correct strain is used. One of the methods is serotyping, that is, identifying a bacterium by the response it triggers in the immune system when it reaches the blood. *E. coli* Nissle 1917 has a serotype O6:K5:H1.

Serotypes that are part of the O6 group show "a broad spectrum of virulence". This means that there are some *E. coli* strains that are similar to the Nissle strain and are pathogenic. Some of those pathogenic *E. coli* O6 strains are a common cause of urinary infections.[3]

As some bacteria pass genetic material to other bacteria, it is possible that the Nissle strain could gain pathogenic characteristics from other *E. coli* strains present in the microflora. Ardeypharm state, however, that among the nine safety aspects of the Nissle strain, there is the characteristic of "no uptake of external pathogenic DNA". In other words, *E. coli* Nissle 1917 will not accept potentially harmful genetic material from other strains of *E. coli* bacteria.

Lactobacilli

With so many different species and strains of lactobacilli used in probiotics, it is reasonable to ask whether any of them are dangerous.

In a review of the medical literature, Jay Sussman and colleagues found 24 cases of endocarditis (inflammation of the lining of the heart) caused by lactobacilli. Six of these patients died.

It should be noted that almost all of the 24 patients already had heart disease and three-quarters had had dental work prior to developing endocarditis. It may be assumed that lactobacilli normally present in the mouth entered the blood-stream at the time of the dental work, and that the patients' immune systems were unable to overcome them.[4]

The Sussman review also found evidence of a handful of cases of other infections caused by lactobacilli, almost certainly from the patients' own gut microflora.

A more recent review reported several cases of bacteraemia (bacteria in the blood) caused by lactobacilli, although it should be noted that the people affected also had other diseases.[5]

Do probiotic products cause lactobacillus infection?

In 1995, a European Union-sponsored workshop reviewed the safety of all lactic acid bacteria (LAB), including lactobacilli, and the specialist microbiologists concluded that, "In most cases of infection the organism appears to have come from the patient's own microflora. No cases have been reported in people working with LAB and routinely exposed to very high numbers, such as those in the starter culture industry. No cases have been linked to the consumption of fermented foods or probiotics".[6]

In 1999, however, a group of Finnish doctors and scientists reported the case of a 74-year-old woman with a history of hypertension and diabetes, who had developed a liver abscess caused by a bacterium indistinguishable from *L. rhamnosus* GG. She recovered after receiving antibiotics for six weeks. She had been taking about half a litre a day of dairy drinks containing *L. rhamnosus* GG to relieve abdominal discomfort during the four months prior to the start of her symptoms.

The Finnish team believed that this was the first reported case of a lactobacillus probiotic product causing a severe infection.[7]

In the same year, another case was reported of a 67-year-old man who developed endocarditis after tooth extraction. The *L. rhamnosus* strain responsible was indistinguishable from the *L. rhamnosus* in the probiotic capsule the man "was accustomed to chewing". This is an unusual way of consuming a capsule and is not recommended.[8]

Putting the information in context

It is important to put this information in context.

Surveys of endocarditis have indicated that lactic acid bacteria (excluding enterococcus) caused the disease only in approximately one case in 1,000.[9]

In Southern Finland two studies were undertaken of bacteraemia cases over a 4- and a 6-year period. In one study only eight out of 3,317 cases were caused by lactobacilli, and in the other study only 12 out of 5,192. None of the 20 lactobacilli cases were related to food, dairy or pharmaceutical strains.[10]

Thus, out of a large number of cases of bacterial infection of the blood, only a tiny proportion was caused by lactobacilli, and none were from probiotic products.

Furthermore, based on Finnish data, it has been reported that "No increase in the number of cases of Lactobacillus bacteraemia has been detected in a national surveillance program, even though the consumption of probiotics has increased several fold during the period of observation".[11]

On the very rare occasions when lactobacilli do cause infection, almost exclusively from the microflora rather than from probiotics, treatment is straightforward as there are plenty of safe antibiotics available to which they are sensitive.[10]

A review of the safety of lactobacilli and other lactic acid bacteria concluded that "large amount of data from clinical trials or studies in human volunteers … attest to the safety of lactic acid bacteria".[12] Another review reported that "Lactic acid bacteria are ubiquitous and have long been used in the production of a wide range of foods since ancient times without adverse effects in humans".[5]

Is there extra risk for people with IBD?
In their review of the safety of lactic acid bacteria, M. Aguirre and M. D. Collins commented that with lactobacillus infection "Underlying disease or immunosuppression are a common feature in these cases, whereas infection in previously healthy humans is extremely rare".[5] This means that among the very low numbers of people who have developed infections from the body's resident lactobacilli, most had a pre-existing disease or weakened immune system.

As IBD is a disease, and drug treatment involves suppressing the immune function, the risk from lactobacilli may be higher in people with IBD compared with healthy people. Therefore, before deciding to take a probiotic it would be sensible to discuss such issues with your doctor, no matter how miniscule the risk.

Enterococci
Enterococci are the only lactic acid bacteria used as a probiotic about which there have been expressions of concern.

Stig Bengmark reported that hospitals have seen a significant rise in recent years of enterococcal infections acquired by in-patients (especially *Ent. faecium* and *Ent. faecalis*). This cause of hospital-acquired infection is second only in numbers to pathogenic *Escherichia coli*. From 1992 to 1994, enterococci made up 30.6 per cent of all surgical intensive care bacteraemia episodes at John Hopkins institutions in Baltimore.[13]

Aguirre and Collins referred to cases of meningitis, endocarditis, bacteraemia and urinary tract infections in which enterococci were the primary pathogens. Also, they described enterococci as being resistant to a wide variety of antibiotics and having a tendency to acquire and disseminate resistance genes. They concluded that the evidence casts doubt on the wisdom of using enterococci as probiotics.[5]

Despite this concern, it must be stressed that there have been no recorded cases of anyone developing disease as a result of taking a probiotic containing enterococcus bacteria.

Furthermore, Tiina Mattila-Sandholm and colleagues pointed out that enterococcal strains are present in many traditional fermented foods without any apparent risk.[14]

Responsibility may lie with the manufacturers of probiotics that contain enterococcal species to provide information on the degree of antibiotic resistance in their strains, as well as evidence of the likelihood that resistance might be passed on to pathogenic bacteria in the microflora. In this way, consumers and health professionals will be better informed.

Bifidobacteria

There have been only a handful of recorded cases of infection by bifidobacteria and these cases did not occur as a result of consuming probiotic products. For example, a baby in Japan developed meningitis caused by *Bifidobacterium breve*. It was a mild infection and was successfully treated by antibiotics. The mother had Behcet's syndrome (a systemic inflammatory disease) and her weakened immunity may have been transferred to the baby via the placenta.[15]

Confidence in the safety of bifidobacteria was strengthened by a study by Shoji Yamazaki and colleagues in which *Bif. longum* was added to germ-free mice. The bifidobacteria soon translocated (crossed from the intestine to the bloodstream) but there was no infection or any harmful effect as a consequence. The translocation also ceased after the fourth week.[16]

In the 1990s two expert group meetings, in the U.S.A. and in Europe, independently of each other concluded that bifidobacteria should be classified as 'Generally Recognised as Safe'.[17]

It is worth noting that bifidobacteria are found in large numbers in the human intestine, and among breast-fed babies they initially constitute up to 90 per cent of the total intestinal bacteria.

Saccharomyces boulardii

There have been no reports of adverse reactions to *Saccharomyces boulardii* product in controlled trials involving more than 2,500 people.[18]

In clinical use, however, a very small number of cases of fungemia (fungal infection of the blood) have been reported. They were easily treated by fungicides. Unlike lactic-acid bacterial infection, which very rarely originates from commercial products, these cases of fungemia do appear to have been associated with *S. boulardii* products.

Confusion with Saccharomyces cerevisiae

Part of the difficulty in deciding which fungal infections have been caused by *S. boulardii* is this particular species' closeness to another yeast, *S. cerevisiae*. Some of the cases of fungemia were identified as being caused by *S. cerevisiae*, although the patients concerned had recently been receiving *S. boulardii*.

There has been a debate as to whether *S. boulardii* is a separate species, or whether it is another strain of *S. cerevisiae*. The most recent genetic analysis suggests that it should be classified as a sub-species of *S. cerevisiae*.

The importance of this debate for people with IBD is that it suggests that some of the rare cases of infection by *S. cerevisiae* may have been caused by *S. boulardii*. Therefore, the risks associated with the boulardii yeast may be slightly higher than had been thought previously.

Michael McCullogh and colleagues, who examined three commercial products of boulardii, described the yeasts as having 'moderate virulence'. Although they acknowledged recent studies confirming the safety of the boulardii yeast, the McCullogh team advised caution in the clinical use of this yeast in patients with weakened immune systems.[19]

As a significant number of the reported cases of fungemia were found in patients with vascular catheters (tube placed directly into blood vessel) it has been suspected that some of the boulardii product powder may have drifted in the air and gained access to the bloodstream through the opening in the skin. This does not constitute a risk for routine home consumption of this yeast probiotic.[20]

Another reassuring factor is that *S. cerevisiae* is the species of yeast used in wine, beer and bread production. As the two yeasts appear to have a similar virulence, and baker's yeast has been used safely in households for centuries, *S. boulardii* should be seen as having a similar safety profile.

Bacillus subtilis

Bacillus subtilis is a spore-producing soil-based bacterium that is sometimes used in probiotic products. A recent review reported seven cases of infection arising from the consumption of *B. subtilis* probiotic products.[21]

The pathogenic potential of *B. subtilis* is low, but it appears that in a few people with severely weakened immune systems infections may develop.[22]

Individual risk

Putting a figure on the risk to health for an individual is almost impossible, because every individual on the planet is unique. Although stringent testing of drugs before they are licensed tell us the proportion of people who are likely to react badly to them, it is not possible to predict which individuals will experience adverse reactions to the drugs. As probiotics are classified as food rather than as drugs, there is less information available on their safety.

Philippe Marteau summarised the current evidence on the safety of probiotics as showing that "although a zero risk does not exist, the risk is extremely low".[8]

Appendix summary

- The human intestinal microflora normally cause no infections, but some can cause disease if the body is weak or vulnerable.

- People with IBD have an increased risk of infection from external pathogens and opportunistic microflora, because there may be sores on the intestine wall that makes it easier for the pathogens to become established, and anti-inflammatory medication prescribed for IBD may weaken the body's immune system.

- Probiotic products carry very little extra risk, because usually they contain bacteria discovered in human intestines, and therefore are unlikely to act as pathogens. Additionally, probiotic bacteria do not become established in the gut or remain long in the intestines.

- The manufacturers of *E. coli* Nissle 1917 use four different methods to check that the correct strain is present in the Mutaflor product. The company also states that *E. coli* Nissle 1917 does not accept genetic material from pathogenic bacteria.

- Lactobacilli have been known to cause a very small amount of disease (for example, endocarditis, bacteraemia). In virtually every case this appears to have arisen from the microflora rather than a probiotic product.

- Data from Finland showed that during a period when consumption of probiotics increased several-fold, there was no increase in bacteraemia cases.

- There are concerns about the safety of enterococci bacteria and whether they are suitable for probiotic products. However, there are no known cases of disease developing from enterococci in a probiotic.

- The risk from bifidobacteria products appears to be as low as that for products containing lactobacilli.

- There have been a small number of fungal infections of the blood caused by *Saccharomyces boulardii,* but this may have been the result of contaminated vascular catheters.

- The soil-based bacterium *Bacillus subtilis*, used as a probiotic, has caused infections in a small number of individuals with weakened immune systems. Its general pathogenic potential is low, however.
- Although the risk from probiotics is not zero, it is extremely low.

References

Chapter 2. The History of Probiotics

1. Lilly, D. M., and R. H. Stillwell, 1965. Probiotics: growth promoting factors produced by microorganisms. *Science* 47: 747-748.

2. Fuller, R. 1989. Probiotics in man and animals. *Journal of Applied Bacteriology* 66:365-378.

3. Newman, James, 2000. Wine. In Kiple, Kenneth and Kriemhild C. Ornelas, eds. *The Cambridge World History of Food*. 730-737. Cambridge: Cambridge University Press.

4. Cantrell, Phillip, 2000. Beer and Ale. In Kiple, Kenneth and Kriemhild C. Ornelas, eds. *The Cambridge World History of Food* 619-625. Cambridge: Cambridge University Press.

5. Bengmark, S., 1998. Ecological control of the gastrointestinal tract. The role of probiotic flora. *Gut* 42: 2-7.

6. Postgate, John, 2000. *Microbes and Man* 18. Cambridge, UK. Cambridge University Press.

7. Hudson, Robert P., 1989. Theory and Therapy: Ptosis, Stasis and Autointoxication. *Bulletin of the History of Medicine* 63: 392-413.

8. Chen, Thomas S. N. and Peter S. Y. Chen, 1989. Intestinal Autointoxication: A Medical Leitmotif. *Journal of Clinical Gastroenterology* 11: 434-441.

9. Medical Press and Circular, 1916. Metchnikoff and Buttermilk. *Journal of the American Medical Association* 67: 939.

10. de Kruif, Paul, 1926. *Microbe Hunters* 201-227. San Diego, USA: Harcourt Brace.

11. Kulp, Walter L. and Leo F. Rettger, 1924. Comparative Study of Lactobacillus Acidophilus and Lactobacillus Bulgaricus. *Journal of Bacteriology* 9: 357-394.

12. Fuller, Roy, 1992. History and developments of probiotics. In Fuller, Roy, ed. *Probiotics – The Scientific Basis* 1-8. London: Chapman and Hall.

13. Shortt, C., 1999. The probiotic century: historical and current perspectives. *Trends in Food Science and Technology* 10: 411-417.

14. Cheplin, Harry A. and Leo F. Rettger, 1922. The Therapeutic Application of Lactobacillus Acidophilus. *Abstracts of Bacteriology* 6: 24.

15. Heasman, Michael and Julian Mellentin, 2001. *The Functional Food Revolution*. London: Earthscan Publications.

16. Cummings, John H. and G. T. Macfarlane, 2001. Is there a role for microorganisms? In Jewell, Derek P., Bryan F. Warren and Neil J. Mortensen, eds. *Challenges in Inflammatory Bowel Disease* 42-51. Oxford, UK: Blackwell Science.

17. WHO Scientific Working Party Group 1994. *Monitoring and Management of Bacterial Resistance to Antimicrobial Agents*. Geneva: WHO.

18. Nurmi, E. and M. Rantala, 1973. New Aspects of Salmonella Infection in Broiler Production. *Nature* 241: 210-211.

19. Barrow, Paul A., 1992. Probiotics for Chickens. In Fuller, Roy, ed. *Probiotics – The Scientific Basis* 226–257. London: Chapman and Hall.

20. Fuller, Roy, 1999. Probiotics for Farm Animals. In Tannock, Gerald, ed. *Probiotics: A Critical Review* 15-22. Wymondham: Horizon Scientific Press.

Chapter 3. IBD, Bacteria and Inflammation

1. Savage, Dwayne C., 1977. Microbial Ecology of the Gastrointestinal Tract. *Annual Review of Microbiology* 31: 107-133.

2. Berg, Rodney D., 1996. The indigenous gastrointestinal microflora. *Trends in Microbiology* 4: 430-435.

3. Macfarlane, G.T., and S. Macfarlane, 1997. Human Colonic Microbiota: Ecology, Physiology and Metabolic Potential of Intestinal Bacteria. *Scandinavian Journal of Gastroenterology* 32 Suppl. 222: 3-9.

4. Faubion, William A. and William J. Sandborn, 2000. Probiotic Therapy with E. Coli for Ulcerative Colitis: Taking the Good with the Bad. *Gastroenterology* 118: 630-635.

5. Cummings, John H. and G. T. Macfarlane, 2001. Is there a role for microorganisms? In Jewell, Derek P., Bryan F. Warren, and Neil J. Mortensen, eds. *Challenges in Inflammatory Bowel Disease* 42-51. Oxford: Blackwell Science.

6. McCracken, Vance J. and H. Rex Gaskins, 1999. Probiotics and the Immune System. In Tannock, Gerald ed. *Probiotics: A Critical Review* 85-111. Wymondham: Horizon Scientific Press.

7. Sompayrac, Lauren, 1999. *How the Immune System Works*. Massachusetts, USA: Blackwell Science.

8. Erikson, Kent L. and Neil E. Hubbard 2000. Probiotic Immunomodulation in Health and Disease. *Journal of Nutrition* 130: 403S-409S.

9. Shanahan, Fergus, 2001. Inflammatory Bowel Disease: Immunodiadnostics, Immunotherapeutics, and Ecotherapeutics. *Gastroenterology* 120: 622-635.

Chapter 4. Probiotics for IBD: Evidence of Benefit

1. Schultz, Michael and R. Balfour Sartor, 2000. Probiotics and Inflammatory Bowel Diseases. *American Journal of Gastroenterology* 95 Suppl. 1: S19-S21.

2. Faubion, William A. and William J. Sandborn, 2000. Probiotic Therapy with *E. Coli* for Ulcerative Colitis: Taking the Good with the Bad. *Gastroenterology* 118: 630-635.

3. Cummings, John H. and G. T. Macfarlane, 2001. Is there a role for microorganisms? In Jewell, Derek P., Bryan F. Warren, and Neil J. Mortensen, eds. *Challenges in Inflammatory Bowel Disease* 42-51. Oxford: Blackwell Science.

4. Campieri, Massimo and Paolo Gionchetti, 1999. Probiotics in Inflammatory Bowel Disease: New Insight to Pathogenesis or a Possible Therapeutic Alternative? *Gastroenterology* 116: 1246-1260.

5. Kennedy, R. J., S. J. Kirk and K.R. Gardiner, 2000. Promotion of a Favourable Gut Flora in Inflammatory Bowel Disease. *Journal of Parenteral and Enteral Nutrition* 24: 189-195.

6. Hamilton-Miller, Jeremy M.T., 2001. A review of trials of probiotics in the management of inflammatory bowel disease. *Infectious Disease Review* 3: 83-87.

7. Shanahan, Fergus, 2000. Probiotics and Inflammatory Bowel Disease: Is there a Scientific Rationale? *Inflammatory Bowel Diseases* 6: 107-115.

8. Katz, Jeffrey A. and Claudio Fiocchi 2001. Probiotic Therapy for IBD. *Inflammatory Bowel Disease Monitor* 4: 106-111.

9. Gionchetti, P., F. Rizzello, A. Ferrieri, A. Venturi, C. Brignola, M. Ferretti, S. Perruzzo, M. Miglioli and M. Campieri, 1999. Rifamixin in Patients with Moderate or Severe Ulcerative Colitis Refractory to Steroid-Treatment: A Double-Blind, Placebo-Controlled Trial. *Digestive Diseases and Sciences* 44: 1220-1221.

10. Rutgeerts, P., K. Goboes, M. Peeters, M. Hiele, F. Penninckx, R. Aerts, R. Kerremans and G. Vantrappen, 1991. Effect of faecal stream diversion on recurrence of Crohn's disease in neoterminal ileum. *The Lancet* 338: 771-774.

11. D'Haens, G. R., K. Geboes, M. Peeters, F. Baert, F. Penninckx and P. Rutgeerts, 1998. Early Lesions of Recurrent Crohn's Disease Caused by Infusion of Intestinal Contents in Excluded Ileum. *Gastroenterology* 114: 262-267.

12. Sellon, R. K., S. Tonkonogy, M. Schultz, L. A. Dieleman, W. Grenther, E. Balish, D. M. Rennick and R. B. Sartor, 1998. Resident Enteric Bacteria are Necessary for Development of Spontaneous Colitis and Immune System Activation in Interleukin-10-Deficient Mice. *Infection and Immunity* 66: 5224-5231.

13. Giaffer, M. H., C. D. Holdsworth and B. I. Duerden 1991. The assessment of faecal flora in patients with inflammatory bowel disease by a simplified bacteriological technique. *Journal of Medical Microbiology* 35: 238-243.

14. Fabia R., A. Ar'Rajab, M-L. Johansson, R. Andersson, R. Willen, B. Jeppsson, G. Molin and S. Bengmark, 1993. Impairment of Bacterial Flora in Human Ulcerative Colitis and Experimental Colitis in the Rat. *Digestion* 54: 248-255.

15. Swidsinski, A., A. Ladhoff, A. Pernthaler, S. Swidsinski, V. Loening-Baucke, M. Ortner, J. Weber, U. Hoffman, S. Schreiber, M. Dietel and H. Lochs, 2002. Mucosal Flora in Inflammatory Bowel Disease. *Gastroenterology* 122: 44-54.

16. Rath, Heiko C., Kenneth H. Wilson and R. Balfour Sartor 1999. Differential Induction of Colitis and Gastritis in HLA-B27 Transgenic Rats Selectively Colonised with *Bacteroides vulgatus* or *Escherichia coli*. *Infection and Immunity* 67: 2969-2974.

17. Wells, C. L., E. M. A. van de Westerlo, R. P. Jechorek, B. A. Feltis, T. D. Wilkins and S. L. Erlandsen, 1996. *Bacteroides fragilis* Enterotoxin Modulates Epithelial Permeability and Bacterial Internalization by HT-29 Enterocytes. *Gastroenterology* 110: 1429-1437.

18. Fabia, R., A. Ar'rajab, M-L. Johansson, R. Willen, R. Andersson, G. Molin, and S. Bengmark, 1993. The Effect of Exogenous Administration of Lactobacillus reuteri R2LC and Oat Fiber on Acetic Acid-Induced Colitis in the Rat. *Scandinavian Journal of Gastroenterology* 28: 155-162.

19. Mao Y, S. Nobaek, B. Kasravi, D. Adawi, U. Stenram, G. Molin and B. Jeppsson, 1996. The Effects of Lactobacillus Strains and Oat Fiber on Methotrexate-Induced Enterocolitis in Rats. *Gastroenterology* 111: 334-344.

20. Madsen, K. L., J. S. Doyle, L. D. Jewell, M. M. Tavernini, and R. N. Fedorak, 1999. Lactobacillus Species Prevent Colitis in Interleukin 10 Gene–Deficient Mice. *Gastroenterology* 116: 1107-1114.

21. Madsen, K., A. Cornish, P. Soper, C. McKaigney, H. Jijon, C. Yachimec, J. Doyle, L. Jewell and C. de Simone, 2001. Probiotic Bacteria Enhance Murine and Human Intestinal Epithelial Barrier Function. *Gastroenterology* 121: 580-591.

22. Sartor, R. B., 1997. Review article: How relevant to human inflammatory bowel disease are current animal models of intestinal inflammation? *Alimentary Pharmacology and Therapeutics* 11 (Suppl.): 89-97.

23. Bennet, Justin D. and Mark Brinkman, 1989. Treatment of Ulcerative Colitis by Implantation of Normal Colonic Flora. *The Lancet* 1: 164.

24. Kruis, W., E. Schutz, P. Fric. B. Fixa, G. Judmaier and M. Stolte 1997. Double-blind comparison of an oral Escherichia coli preparation and mesalazine in maintaining remission of ulcerative colitis. *Alimentary Pharmacology and Therapeutics* 11: 853-858.

25. Rembacken, B. J., A. M. Snelling, P. M.Hawkey, D. M. Chalmers and A. T. R. Axon 1999. Non-pathogenic Escherichia coli versus mesalazine for the treatment of ulcerative colitis: a random trial. *Lancet* 354: 635-639.

26. Kruis, W., P. Fric and M. Stolte, 2001. Maintenance of Remission in Ulcerative Colitis is Equally Effective with Escherichia coli Nissle 1917 and with Standard Mesalamine. *Gastroenterology* 120 Suppl. 1: A127 (Abstr. 680).

27. Malchow, Helmut A., 1997. Crohn's Disease and Escherichia Coli. *Journal of Clinical Gastroenterology* 25: 653-658.

28. Venturi, A., P. Gionchetti, F. Rizzello, R. Johansson, E. Zucconi, P. Brigidi, D. Matteuzzi and M. Campieri, 1999. Impact on the composition of the fecal flora by a new probiotic preparation: preliminary data on maintenance treatment of patients with ulcerative colitis. *Alimentary Pharmacology and Therapeutics* 13: 1103-1108.

29. Gionchetti, P., F. Rizzello, A. Venturi, P. Brigidi, D. Mattuezi, G. Bazzocchi, G. Poggioli, M. Miglioli and M. Campieri, 2000. Oral Bacteriotherapy as Maintenance Treatment in Patients with Chronic Pouchitis: A Double-Blind, Placebo-Controlled Trial. *Gastroenterology* 119: 305-309.

30. Guslandi, M., G. Mezzi, M. Sorghi, and P. A. Testoni, 2000. Saccharomyces boulardii in Maintenance Treatment of Crohn's Disease. *Digestive Diseases and Sciences* 45: 1462-1464.

Chapter 5. Specific Species and Strains

1. Hamilton-Miller, Jeremy M.T., 2001. A review of trials of probiotics in the management of inflammatory bowel disease. *Infectious Disease Review* 3: 83-87.

2. Tannock, Gerald W., 1999. Modification of the normal microflora. In Tannock, G. W., ed. *Medical Importance of the Normal Microflora* 487-506. Netherlands: Kluwer Academic Publishers.

3. Rembacken, B. J., A. M. Snelling, P. M. Hawkey, D. M. Chalmers and A. T. R.Axon 1999. Non-pathogenic Escherichia coli versus mesalazine for the treatment of ulcerative colitis: a random trial. *Lancet* 354: 635-639.

4. Gibson, G.R, and X. Wang, 1994. Regulatory effects of bifidobacteria on the growth of other colonic bacteria. *Journal of Applied Bacteriology* 77: 412-420.

5. Cooke, E. Mary, 1968. Properties of strains of Escherichia coli isolated from the faeces of patients with ulcerative colitis, patients with acute diarrhoea and normal persons. *Journal of Pathology and Bacteriology* 95: 101-113.

6. Giaffer, M. H., C. D. Holdsworth and B. I. Duerden 1992. Virulence properties of Escherichia coli strains isolated from patients with inflammatory bowel disease. *Gut* 33: 646-650.

7. Fuller, R., 1989. Probiotics in man and animals. *Journal of Applied Bacteriology* 66:365-378.

8. Kennedy, R. J., S. J. Kirk, and K. R. Gardiner, 2000. Promotion of a Favourable Gut Flora in Inflammatory Bowel Disease. *Journal of Parenteral and Enteral Nutrition* 24: 189-195.

9. Gilliland, Stanley E., 1990. Health and nutritional benefits from lactic acid bacteria. *FEMS Microbiology Reviews* 87: 175-188.

10. Bengmark, S., 1998. Ecological control of the gastrointestinal tract. The role of probiotic flora. *Gut* 42: 2-7.

11. Mack, D. R., S. Michail, S. Wei, L. McDougall and M. A. Hollingsworth, 1999. Probiotics inhibit enteropathogenic E. coli adherence in vitro by inducing intestinal mucin gene expression. *American Journal of Physiology* 276: G941-G950.

12. Ballongue, Jean, 1998. Bifidobacteria and Probiotic Action. In Salminen, Seppo, and Atte von Wright, eds., *Lactic Acid Bacteria* 519-587. New York: Marcel Dekker.

13. Macfarlane, G. T., G. R. Gibson, B. S. Drasar and J. H. Cummings, 1995. Metabolic significance of the gut microflora. In Whitehead, R., ed. *Gastrointestinal and Oesophagal Pathology* 249-274. Edinburgh: Churchill Livingstone.

14. Bernet, M-F., D. Brassart, J-R. Neeser and A. L. Servin, 1993. Adhesion of Human Bifidobacterial Strains to Cultured Human Intestinal Epithelial Cells and Inhibition of Enteropathogen–Cell Ineractions. *Applied and Environmental Microbiology* 59: 4121-4128.

15. Mogensen, Gunnar, 2000. Bifidobacteria. In Gibson, G. and F. Angus, eds., *LFRA Ingredients Handbook – Prebiotics and Probiotics* 85-115. Leatherhead: LFRA.

16. Periti, P. and F. Tonelli, 2001. Preclinical and Clinical Pharmacology of Biotherapeutic Agents: Saccharomyces boulardii. *Journal of Chemotherapy* 13: 473-493.

17. Summers, R. W., J. Urban, D. Elliott, K. Qadir, R. Thompson and J. Weinstock, 1999. Th2 conditioning by Trichuris suis appears safe and effective in modifying the mucosal immune response in inflammatory bowel disease. *Gastrenterology* 116: A828 (abstr.).

18. Shanahan, Fergus, 2000. Probiotics and Inflammatory Bowel Disease: Is there a Scientific Rationale? *Inflammatory Bowel Diseases* 6: 107-115.

19. Buydens, P. and S. Debeuckelaere, 1996. Efficacy of SF68 in the Treatment of Acute Diarrhoea. *Scandinavian Journal of Gastroenterology* 31: 887-891.

20. Hamilton-Miller, J. M. T. and S. Shah, 1998. Benefits and Risks of Enterococcus faecium as a Probiotic. In Sadler, M. J. and M. Saltmarsh, eds. *Functional Foods – The Consumer, the Products and the Evidence* 20-24. Cambridge: The Royal Society of Chemistry.

21. Salminen, S., A. von Wright, L. Morelli, P. Marteau, D. Brassart, W. M. de Vos, R. Fonden, M. Saxelin, K. Collins, G. Mogensen, S-E. Birkeland and T. Mattila-Sandholm, 1998. Demonstration of safety of probiotics – a review. *International Journal of Food Microbiology* 44: 93-106.

Chapter 6. *Prebiotics:* What are they?

1. Gibson, Glenn and Marcel B. Roberfroid, 1995. Dietary Modulation of the Human Colonic Microbiota: Introducing the Concept of Prebiotics. *Journal of Nutrition* 125: 1401-1412.

2. Macfarlane, G.T., and S. Macfarlane, 1999. Human Colonic Microbiota: Ecology, Physiology and Metabolic Potential of Intestinal Bacteria. *Scandinavian Journal of Gastroenterology* 32 Suppl. 222: 3-9.

3. Crittenden, Ross, 1999. *Prebiotics*. In Tannock, Gerald, ed. *Probiotics: A Critical Review* 141-156. Wymondham: Horizon Scientific Press.

4. Ballongue J., C. Schumann and P. Quignon, 1997. Effects of Lactulose and Lactitol on Colonic Microflora and Enzymic Activity. *Scandinavian Journal of Gastroenterology* 32 Suppl. 222: 41-44.

5. Bouhnik Y., B. Flourie, M. Riottot, N. Bisetti, M. Gailing, A. Guibert, F. Bornet and J. Rambaud, 1996. Effects of fructo-oligosaccharide ingestion on fecal bifidobacteria and selected metabolic indexes of colon carcinogenesis in healthy humans. *Nutrition and Cancer* 26: 21-29.

6. Van Loo, J., J. Cummings, N. Delzenne, H. Englyst, A. Franck, M. Hopkins, N. Kok, G. Macfarlane, D. Newton, M. Quigley, M. Roberfroid, T. van Vliet and E. van den Heuvel. Functional food properties of non-digestible oligosaccharides: a consensus report from the ENDO project. *British Journal of Nutrition* 81: 121-132.

7. Zopf, David and Stephen Roth, 1996. Oligosaccharide anti-infective agents. *Lancet* 347: 1017-1021.

8. Gibson, Glenn, Robert A. Rastall and Marcel B. Roberfroid, 1999. *Prebiotics*. In Gibson, Glenn and Marcel B. Roberfroid, eds. *Colonic Microbiota, Nutrition and Health* 101-124. Netherlands: Kluwer Academic Publishers.

9. Madsen, L., J. S. Doyle, L. D. Jewell, M. M. Tavernini, and R. N. Fedorak, 1999. Lactobacillus Species Prevent Colitis in Interleukin 10 Gene–Deficient Mice. *Gastroenterology* 116: 1107-1114.

10. Videla, S., J. Vilaseca, M. Antolin, A. Garcia-Lafuente, F. Guarner, E. Crespo, J. Casalots, A. Salas and J. R. Malagelada, 2001. Dietary Inulin Improves Distal Colitis Induced by Dextran Sodium Sulfate in the Rat. *American Journal of Gastroenterology* 96: 1486-1493.

11. Teramoto, F., K. Rokutan, Y. Kawakami, Y. Fujimura, J. Uchida, K. Oku, M. Oka and M. Yoneyama 1996. Effect of lactosucrose on fecal microflora in patients with chronic inflammatory bowel disease. *Journal of Gastroenterology* 31: 33-39.

12. Welters, C., E. Heineman, F. Thunnissen, A. van den Bogaard, P. Soeters and C. Baeten, 2002. Effect of Dietary Inulin Supplementation on Inflammation of Pouch Mucosa in Patients with Ileal Pouch-Anal Anastamosis. *Diseases of the Colon and Rectum* 45: 621-627.

13. Pedersen, Annette, Brittmarie Sandstrom and Johan M. M. Van Amelsvoort, 1997. The effect of ingestion of inulin on blood lipids and gastrointestinal symptoms in healthy females. *British Journal of Nutrition* 78: 215-222

14. Molis, C., B. Flourie, F. Ouarne, M-F. Gailing, S. Lartigue, A. Guibert, F. Bornet and J-P. Galmiche, 1996. Digestion, excretion and energy value of fructooligosaccharides in healthy humans. *American Journal of Clinical Nutrition* 62: 324-328.

Chapter 7. Specific *Prebiotics*

1. Van Loo, J., J. Cummings, N. Delzenne, H. Englyst, A. Franck, M. Hopkins, N. Kok, G. Macfarlane, D. Newton, M. Quigley, M. Roberfroid, T. van Vliet and E. van den Heuvel, 1999. Functional food properties of non-digestible oligosaccharides: a consensus report from the ENDO project. *British Journal of Nutrition* 81: 121-132.

2. Buddington R. K., C. H. Williams, S-C. Chen and S. A. Witherley, 1996. Dietary supplement of neosugar alters the fecal flora and decreases activities of reactive enzymes in human subjects. *American Journal of Clinical Nutrition* 63: 709-716.

3. Teramoto, F., K. Rokutan, Y. Kawakami, Y. Fujimura, J. Uchida, K. Oku, M. Oka and M. Yoneyama 1996. Effect of lactosucrose on fecal microflora in patients with chronic inflammatory bowel disease. *Journal of Gastroenterology* 31: 33-39.

4. Moshfegh, A. J., J. E. Friday, J. P. Goldman, and J. K. C. Ahuja, 1999. Presence of Inulin and Oligofructose in the Diets of Americans. *Journal of Nutrition* 129: 1407S-1411S.

5. Crittenden, Ross, 1999. Prebiotics, 141-156. In Tannock, Gerald, ed. *Probiotics: A Critical Review*, Wymondham, UK: Horizon Scientific Press.

6. Roberfroid, Marcel B., Jan A. E. Van Loo, and Glenn R. Gibson, 1998. The Bifidogenic Nature of Chicory Inulin and Its Hydrolysis Products. *Journal of Nutrition* 128: 11-19.

7. Murphy, Olive, 2001. Non-polyol low-digestible carbohydrates: food applications and functional benefits. *British Journal of Nutrition* 85 Suppl. 1: 26-31.

8. Gibson, G.R., E.R. Beatty, X. Wang, and J.H. Cummings, 1995. Selective Stimulation of Bifidobacteria in the Human Colon by Oligofructose and Inulin. *Gastroenterology* 108: 975-982.

9. Kleeson, B., B. Sykura, H-J. Zunft, and M. Blaut, 1997. Effects of inulin and lactose on fecal microflora microbial activity, and bowel habit in elderly constipated patients. *American Journal of Clinical Nutrition* 65: 1397-1402.

10. Slavin, Joanne, 1999. Dietary Fibre and Non-Digestible Oligosaccharides, 125-147. In Gibson G.R., and M.B. Roberfroid, eds. *Colonic Microbiota, Nutrition and Health*, Netherlands: Kluwer Academic Publishers.

11. Ballongue J., C. Schumann, and P. Quignon, 1997. Effects of Lactulose and Lactitol on Colonic Microflora and Enzymic Activity. *Scandinavian Journal of Gastroenterology* 32 Suppl 222: 41-44.

12. Madsen, L., J. S. Doyle, L. D. Jewell, M. M. Tavernini, and R. N. Fedorak, 1999. Lactobacillus Species Prevent Colitis in Interleukin 10 Gene–Deficient Mice. *Gastroenterology* 116: 1107-1114.

13. Kravtchenko, T. P., 1998. Acacia Gum – A Natural Soluble Fibre. In Sadler, M. J., and M. Saltmarsh, eds. *Functional Foods – The Consumer, the Products and the Evidence* 38-46. Cambridge: The Royal Society of Chemistry.

14. Rycroft C. E., M. R. Jones, G.R. Gibson and R. A. Rastall, 2001. A comparative *in vitro* evaluation of the fermentation properties of prebiotic oligosaccharides. *Journal of Applied Microbiology* 91: 878-887.

15. McBain A. J. and G. T. Macfarlane, 2001. Modulation of genotoxic enzyme activities by non-digestible oligosaccharide metabolism in in-vitro human gut bacterial gut ecosystems. *Journal of Medical Microbiology* 50: 833-842.

16. Gibson, Glenn, Robert A. Rastall, and Marcel B. Roberfroid, 1999. Prebiotics, 101-124. In Gibson, Glenn and Marcel B. Roberfroid, eds. *Colonic Microbiota, Nutrition and Health*, Netherlands: Kluwer Academic Publishers.

17. Videla, S., J. Vilaseca, M. Antolin, A. Garcia-Lafuente, F. Guarner, E. Crespo, J. Casalots, A. Salas and J. R. Malagelada, 2001. Dietary Inulin Improves Distal Colitis Induced by Dextran Sodium Sulfate in the Rat. *American Journal of Gastroenterology* 96: 1486-1493.

18. Gibson, Glenn and Marcel B. Roberfroid, 1995. Dietary Modulation of the Human Colonic Microbiota: Introducing the Concept of Prebiotics. *Journal of Nutrition* 125: 1401-1412.

Chapter 8. Other benefits of Probiotics

1. Marteau, P. R., M. de Vrese, C. J. Cellier and J. Schrezenmeier, 2001. Protection from gastrointestinal diseases with the use of probiotics. *American Journal of Clinical Nutrition* 73: 430S-436S.

2. Rolfe, Rial D., 2000. The Role of Probiotic Cultures in the Control of Gastrointestinal Health. *Journal of Nutrition* 130:396S-402S.

3. Marteau, Philippe R., 2002. Probiotics in Clinical Conditions. *Clinical Reviews in Allergy and Immunology* 22: 255-273.

4. Elmer, G. W., C. M. Surawicz and L. V. McFarland, 1996. Biotherapeutic Agents. *Journal of the American Medical Association (JAMA)* 275: 870-876.

5. Madsen, Karen L., 2001. The use of probiotics in gastrointestinal disease. *Canadian Journal of Gastroenterology* 15: 817-822.

6. Asahara, T., K. Nomoto, K. Shimuzu, M. Watanuki and R. Tanaka, 2001. Increased resistance of mice to Salmonella enterica serovar Typhimurium infection by symbiotic administration of Bifidobacteria and transgalactosylated oligosaccharides. *Journal of Applied Microbiology* 91: 985-996.

7. Pathmakanthan, S., S. Meance and C. A. Edwards, 2000. Probiotics: A Review of Human Studies to Date and Methodological Approaches. *Microbial Ecology in Health and Disease* Suppl. 2: 10-30.

8. Den Hond, Elly, Benny Geypens and Yvo Ghoos, 2000. Effect of High Performance Chicory Inulin on Constipation. *Nutrition Research* 20: 731-736.

9. Forbes, Alastair, 1997. *Clinicians' Guide to Inflammatory Bowel Disease* 213-236. London: Chapman and Hall.

10. Dugas, B., A. Mercenier, I. Lenoir-Wijnkoop, C. Arnaud, N. Dugas and E. Postaire, 1999. Immunity and Probiotics. *Immunology Today* 20: 387-390.

11. Boutron, M-C., J. Faivre, P. Marteau, C. Couillault, P. Senesse and V. Quiport, 1996. Calcium, phosphorus and vitamin D, dairy products and colorectal carcinogenesis: a French case-control study. *British Journal of Cancer* 74: 145-151.

12. Wollowski, Ingrid, Gerhard Rechkemmer and Beatrice L. Pool-Zobel, 2001. Protective role of probiotics and prebiotics in colon cancer. *American Journal of Clinical Nutrition* 73: 451S-455S.

13. Brady, Linda J., Daniel D. Gallagher and Frank. F. Busta, 2000. The Role of Probiotic Cultures in the Prevention of Colon Cancer. *Journal of Nutrition* 130: 410S-414S.

14. Buddington, Karyl K., Jillian B. Donahoo, and Randal K. Buddington, 2002. Dietary Oligofructose and Inulin Protect Mice from Enteric and Systemic Pathogens and Tumor Inducers. *Journal of Nutrition* 132: 472-477.

15. Pool-Zobel, B., J. van Loo, I. Rowland and M. B. Roberfroid, 2002. Experimental evidences on the potential of prebiotic fructans to reduce the risk of colon cancer. *British Journal of Nutrition* 87: S273-S281.

16. Taper, H. S., and M. B. Roberfroid, 2002. Inulin/oligofructose and anticancer therapy. *British Journal of Nutrition* 87: S283-S286.

17. Crittenden, Ross G., 1999. Prebiotics. In Tannock, G.W., ed. *Probiotics: A Critical Review*, 141-156. Wymondham: Horizon Scientific Press.

18. Levy, R., K. R. Jones, W. E. Whitehead, S. I. Feld, N. J. Talley and L. A. Corey, 2001. Irritable Bowel Syndrome in Twins: Heredity and Social Learning Both Contribute to Etiology. *Gastroenterology* 121: 799-804.

19. Hamilton-Miller, J. M. T., 2001. Probiotics in the Management of Irritable Bowel Syndrome: A Review of Clinical Trials. *Microbial Ecology in Health and Disease* 13: 212-216.

20. Niedzielen, Krzysztof, Hubert Kordecki and Bozena Birkenfeld, 2001. A controlled, double-blind, randomised study on the efficacy of *Lactobacillus plantarum* 299v in patients with irritable bowel syndrome. *European Journal of Gastroenterology and Hepatology* 13: 1143-1147.

21. de Vrese, M., A. Stegelmann, B. Richter, S. Fenselau, C. Laue and J. Schrezenmeir, 2001. Probiotics – compensation for lactase insufficiency. *American Journal of Clinical Nutrition* 73: 421S-429S.

22. Szilagyi, A., 2002. Review article: lactose – a potential prebiotic. *Alimentary Pharmacology and Therapeutics* 16: 1591-1602.

23. Newcomer, Albert D. and Douglas B. McGill, 1984. Clinical Importance of Lactose Deficiency. *The New England Journal of Medicine* 310: 42-43.

24. de Vrese, Michael, Birgit Keller and Christian A. Barth, 1992. Enhancement of intestinal hydrolysis of lactose by microbial b-galactosidase of kefir. *British Journal of Nutrition* 67: 67-75.

25. Martini, M. C., E. C. Lerebours, W-J. Lin, S. K. Harlander, N. M. Berrada, J. M. Antoine and D. A. Savaiano, 1991. Strains and species of lactic acid bacteria in fermented milks (yogurts): effect on in vivo lactose digestion. *American Journal of Clinical Nutrition* 54: 1041-1046.

26. Szilagyi, Andrew, Julie Rivard and Kira Fokeeff, 2001. Improved Parameters of Lactose Maldigestion Using Lactulose. *Digestive Diseases and Sciences* 46: 1509-1519.

Chapter 9. Questions and answers on probiotics

1. Gilliland, S. E. and M. L. Speck, 1977. Enumeration and Identity of Lactobacilli in Dietary Products. *Journal of Food Protection* 40: 760-762.

2. Hamilton-Miller, J. M. T., S. Shah and J. T. Winkler, 1999. Public health issues arising from microbiological and labelling quality of foods and supplements containing probiotic microorganisms. *Public Health Nutrition* 2: 223-229.

3. Charteris, W. P., P. M. Kelly, L. Morelli and J. K. Collins, 1998. Development and application of an in vitro methodology to determine the transit tolerance of potentially probiotic Lactobacillus and Bifidobacterium species in the upper human gastrointestinal tract. *Journal of Applied Microbiology* 84: 759-768.

4. van den Merwe, J. P., J. H. Stegeman and M. P. Hazenberg, 1983. The resident faecal flora is determined by genetic characteristics of the host. Implications for Crohn's disease? *Antonie van Leeuwenhoek* 49: 119-124.

5. McCartney, A. L., W. Wenzhi and G. W. Tannock, 1996. Molecular Analysis of the Composition of the Bifidobacterial and Lactobacillus Microflora of Humans. *Applied and Environmental Microbiology* 62: 4608-4613.

6. Tannock, Gerald W., 1997. Probiotic properties of lactic acid bacteria: plenty of scope for fundamental R & D. *Trends in Biotechnology* 15: 270-274.

7. O'Sullivan, Daniel J., 1999. Methods for Analysis of the Intestinal Microflora. In Tannock, Gerald, ed. *Probiotics: A Critical Review* 141-156. Wymondham: Horizon Scientific Press.

8. Mountzouris, K.C., A.L. McCartney and G.R. Gibson, 2002. Intestinal Microflora of human infants and current trends for its nutritional modulation. *British Journal of Nutrition* 87: 405-420.

9. Simakachorn, N., V. Pichaipat, P. Rithipornpaisarn, C. Kongkaew, P. Tongpradit and W. Varavithya, 2000. Clinical evaluation of the Addition of Lyophilized, Heat-Killed Lactobacillus acidophilus LB to Oral Rehydration Therapy in the Treatment of Acute Diarrhea in Children. *Journal of Pediatric Gastroenterology and Nutrition* 30: 68-72.

Appendix 2: Safety of probiotics

1. Tannock, Gerald W., 1999. Modification of the normal microflora. In Tannock, G. W., ed. *Medical Importance of the Normal Microflora* 487-506, Netherlands: Kluwer Academic Publishers.

2. Irrgang, Karl and Ulrich Sonnenborn, 1998. *The historical development of Mutaflor therapy.* Herdecke, Germany: Ardeypharm GmbH.

3. Blum, G., R. Marre and J. Hacker, 1995. Properties of Escherichia coli Strains of Serotype O6. *Infection* 23: 234-236.

4. Sussman, J. I., E. J. Baron, S. M. Goldberg, M. H. Kaplan and R. A. Pizzarello, 1986. Clinical Manifestations and Therapy of Lactobacillus Endocarditis: Report of a Case and Review of Literature. *Review of Infectious Diseases* 8: 771-776.

5. Aguirre, M. and M. D. Collins, 1993. Lactic acid bacteria and human clinical infection. *Journal of Applied Bacteriology* 75: 95-107.

6. Adams, M. R. and P. Marteau 1995. On the safety of lactic acid bacteria from food. *International Journal of Food Microbiology* 27: 263-264.

7. Rautio, M., H. Jousimies-Somer, H. Kauma, I. Pietarinen, M. Saxelin, S. Tynkkynen and M. Koskela, 1999. Liver Abscess Due to a *lactobacillus rhamnosus* Strain Indistinguishable from *L. rhamnosus* Strain GG. *Clinical Infectious Diseases* 28: 1159-1160.

8. Marteau, Philippe R., 2002. Probiotics in Clinical Conditions. *Clinical Reviews in Allergy and Immunology* 22: 255-273.

9. Adams, Martin R., 1999. Safety of industrial lactic acid bacteria. *Journal of Biotechnology* 68: 171-178.

10. Salminen, S., A. von Wright, L. Morelli, P. Marteau, D. Brassart, W. M. de Vos, R. Fonden, M. Saxelin, K. Collins, G. Mogensen, S-E. Birkeland and T. Mattila-Sandholm, 1998. Demonstration of safety of probiotics – a review. *International Journal of Food Microbiology* 44: 93-106.

11. Salminen, Seppo and Heikki Arvilommi, 2002. Safety of Lactobacillus Strains Used as Probiotic Agents. *Clinical Infectious Diseases* 34: 1283-1285.

12. Lee, Y-K., K. Nomoto, S. Salminen and S. L. Gorbach, 1999. Introduction. In Lee *et al.*, *Handbook of Probiotics* 1-22. New York: John Wiley and Sons.

13. Bengmark, S., 1998. Ecological control of the gastrointestinal tract. The role of probiotic flora. *Gut* 42: 2-7.

14. Mattila-Sandholm, Tiina, Jaana Matto and Maria Saarela, 1999. Lactic acid bacteria with health claims – interactions and interference with gastrointestinal flora. *International Dairy Journal* 9: 25-35.

15. Hata, D., A. Yoshida, H. Ohkubo, Y. Mochizuki, Y. Hosoki, R. Tanaka and R. Azuma, 1988. Meningitis Caused by Bifidobacterium in an Infant. *The Pediatric Infectious Disease Journal* 7: 669-671.

16. Ishibashi, Noria and Shoji Yamazaki, 2001. Probiotics and safety. *American Journal of Clinical Nutrition* 73: 465S-470S.

17. Mogensen, Gunnar, 2000. Bifidobacteria. In Gibson, G. and F. Angus, eds. *LFRA Ingredients Handbook Prebiotics and Probiotics.* Leatherhead. LFRA.

18. McFarland, L.V. and P. Bernansconi, 1993. *Saccharomyces boulardii*: A Review of an Innovative Biotherapeutic Agent. *Microbial Ecology in Health and Disease* 6: 157-171.

19. McCullogh, M. J., K. V. Clemons, J. H. McCusker and D. A. Stevens, 1998. Species Identification and Virulence Attributes of *Saccharomyces boulardii* (nom. inval.). *Journal of Clinical Microbiology* 36: 2613-2617.

20. Hennequin, C., C. Kauffmann-Lacroix, A. Jobert, J. P. Viard, C. Ricour, J. L. Jacquemin and P. Berche, 2000. Possible role of catheters in *Saccharomyces boulardii* fungemia. *European Journal of Clinical Microbiology and Infectious Diseases* 19: 16-20.

21. Joint FAO/WHO Working Group, 2002. *Report on Drafting Guidelines for the Evaluation of Probiotics in Food*. Ontario, Canada.

22. Oggioni, M. R., G. Pozzi, P. E. Valensin, P. Galieni and C. Bigazzi, 1998. Recurrent Septicaemia in an Immunocompromised Patient Due to Probiotic Strains of Bacillus subtilis. *Journal of Clinical Microbiology* 36: 325-326.

Index

Symbols
5-ASA 52

A
acacia gum 83
acetic acid 60, 71
acidophilus milk 24, 98
Actimel® 24
adaptive immune system
    41, 103, 106
animal models 48
antibiotic-associated
    diarrhoea (AAD) 88
antibiotic-resistant bacteria
    27, 28, 35
antibiotics 17, 23, 26, 28,
    35, 43, 47
antibodies 42, 106
antigens 106
Ardeypharm 109
autointoxication 22

B
B cells 42, 106
Bacillus subtilis 67, 115
bacteraemia 111
bacteria 29
bacteriocides 39
bacteriocins 56, 59, 61
bacteroides 49, 91
Behcet's syndrome 113
beneficial 29
bifidobacteria 49, 52, 60,
    61, 62, 67, 69, 72, 100,
    113
bifidobacterium 24, 54
Bifidobacterium breve 113
Bio Activia® yoghurt 24
bio-yoghurts 98

C
cancer of the colon 87
children with IBD 101
clinical trials 51
clostridia 80, 82, 91
Clostridium difficile 89

colon cancer 70
colonisation resistance 100
constipation 87, 89
controlled trials 114
corticosteroids 43
Crohn's 33, 34, 37
Cytokines 105

D
Danone 24
diet 12
dietary fibre 70

E
E. coli 49, 55, 67, 80, 110
E. coli Nissle 1917 51, 67
E. coli O157 55
ENDO 72
endocarditis 110
Ent. faecalis 113
Ent. faecium 65, 113
enterococci 65, 67, 112
enterocytes (gut wall cells)
    59
epithelial cells 72
Escherichia coli 49, 51, 113
Escherichia coli Nissle 1917
    ('Mutaflor') 109
eubacteria 91

F
fermented drinks 18
fermented foods 17, 18,
    111
fermented milk 29
fermented milk products
    22, 60, 62, 90
Fleming, Alexander 23
food supplements 99
FOS 81, 85
FOS (oligofructose) 100
fructo-oligosaccharides
    (FOS) 79, 80, 86, 90
fructose 81
functional foods 24, 75
fungemia 114

G
galacto-oligosaccharide 81
gas production 74
gastric acid 41, 103
gastroenteritis 87
genes 11, 37, 43, 102
genus 54, 67
germ-free intestines 48
gluco-oligosaccharides 83
gut bacteria 48, 61, 101,
    108

H
H. pylori 38
heart disease 70
heat 40
Helicobacter pylori 25
helminth worms 64
hydrogen peroxide 59

I
IBD 41, 67, 68, 96, 101
IL10-deficient mice 48
ileo-anal pouch 48
ileo-anal pouches 73
immune system 11, 42, 65,
    101, 112
inflammation 12, 33, 37,
    39, 41, 84, 101, 105
Inflammatory Bowel
    Disease (IBD) 10, 33
infliximab 43, 105
innate immune system 41,
    103
inulin 73, 74, 77, 78, 79,
    80, 81, 85, 86, 90, 91, 100
Irritable Bowel Syndrome
    (IBS) 87, 91
Isomalto-oligosaccharides
    (ISO) 83

K
keffir 19

L
L. acidophilus 24

L. acidophilus LB 102
L. acidophilus NFCO 1748 58
L. bulgaricus 23, 24, 59, 93
L. casei DN-114 001 58
L. casei Shirota 25, 58
L. johnsonii La1 58
L. plantarum 299v 57
L. reuteri 58
L. rhamnosus GG 57, 62, 111
L. salivarius UCC118 57
lactase 92
lactic acid 58, 60, 71
lactic acid bacteria 19, 23, 58, 65, 91, 101, 111
lactic-acid bacteria 24, 65
Lactitol 82
Lactobacilli 110
lactobacilli 49, 52, 57, 61, 67, 100
lactobacillus 24, 54, 57
Lactobacillus acidophilus 24, 54
Lactobacillus delbrueckii subsp. bulgaricus 22
Lactobacillus plantarum 299v 92
Lactobacillus reuteri 73
lactose 62, 82, 83, 92
lactose intolerance 87, 92
lactosucrose 73, 83
Lactosucrose (LS) 83
lactulose 71, 73, 79, 81, 86, 94
Lane, Sir W. Arbuthnot 21, 22
leaky gut 38, 59
low-fibre diet 89
lumen 46
lymph 43
lymph system 42, 106

M
memory cells 106
mesalazine 51
Metchnikoff, Elie 21, 22, 23, 31, 41, 59, 105
microflora 9, 12, 21, 27, 29, 37, 49, 61, 100, 101, 108
milk-based probiotics 98, 99
MMR 38
mucosa 38, 43, 59, 71
mucosal immune system 43

mucosal permeability 38
mucus 41, 43, 67, 103, 104
murine studies 58
Mycobacterium paratuberculosis 38

N
National Institutes of Health 26
NDOs 71, 79, 84, 86
non-digestible oligosaccharides (NDOs) 70, 77
non-IBD diarrhoea 87
non-milk probiotics 99
nutraceuticals 75

O
oligofructose (FOS) 71, 74, 77, 78, 91
oligosaccharides 85
opportunistic pathogens 108

P
pain 39
palatinose 83
Pasteur, Louis 19
pathogens 37
peristalsis 41, 103, 104
phagocyte 104
phagocytes 21, 41, 42, 106
placebo 52
polydextrose 83
pouchitis 47, 52
prebiotics 10, 14, 69
probiotic bacteria 9, 12, 14
probiotic supplements 99
proctitis 54
PROEUHEALTH 66, 68
purgatives 20
pyrodextrin 83

R
randomised controlled trials (RCTs) 11, 88, 92
resistant starch 83
Rettger, Leo F. 23, 24

S
S. thermophilus 93
Saccharomyces boulardii 63, 67, 89, 114
Saccharomyces cerevisiae 114
Salmonella 109

Shirota, Dr Minoru 24
short-chain fatty acids (SCFAs) 59
Sir W. Arbuthnot Lane 23
skin 41, 103, 104
Soyo-oligosaccharides (SOS) 82
species 54, 67
Stasis 20
stoma 40, 47, 80
stomach acid 23, 25, 56, 63, 80, 81, 85, 94, 97, 98, 104
stomach ulcers 25
strain 54, 67
Streptococcus salivarius 52
Streptococcus thermophilus 23, 59
sucrose 80, 83
Swann Committee 27
synbiotics 85, 86

T
T cells 106
T-helper cells 43, 64
the body's defence systems 103
Tissier, Henry 61
Transgalacto-oligosaccharides (TOS) 75, 79, 81, 82, 86
Trichuris suis 67

U
UC 33, 34, 37

V
van Leeuwenhoek, Antoni 19
VSL#3 52, 66, 68

W
white blood cells 39, 41, 43, 104
World Health Organisation (WHO) 28

X
Xylo-oligosaccharides (XOS) 83

Y
Yakult 25
yoghurt 19, 59, 90, 93, 99
yoghurts 22, 25